KU-657-378

Foreword

It is a pleasure to introduce this Neurological Compendium prepared by CONCAH which is a voluntary organisation concerned with the complexities of providing continuing care at home for people with a range of conditions. Neurological disorders account for a large proportion of these.

The compendium is designed to make information about some common and some rare disorders easily accessible and to help health professionals respond appropriately to the needs of people who suffer from these disorders.

Changes in the National Health Service in recent years have included the adoption of the purchaser/provider principle and greater emphasis on accountability for the services provided. Some have feared that this might threaten those caring functions of professionals which are difficult to measure and to price. In the face of this challenge, the British Medical Association, during my presidency, held a conference to review the 'core values' of the medical profession. This brought together all the Presidents of the Royal Medical Colleges, the Conference of Deans and senior officers in the Association. The conference reaffirmed the importance of the profession's ancient virtues distilled over time, summarising these as commitment, confidentiality, compassion, caring and competence, linked to a spirit of enquiry and advocacy.

CONCAH brings together all these core values in its approach to disability. It goes far beyond this however because it acknowledges the importance of team care and the vital role played by the disabled themselves and their carers. Through workshops

Neurological compendium

A resource book for general practice

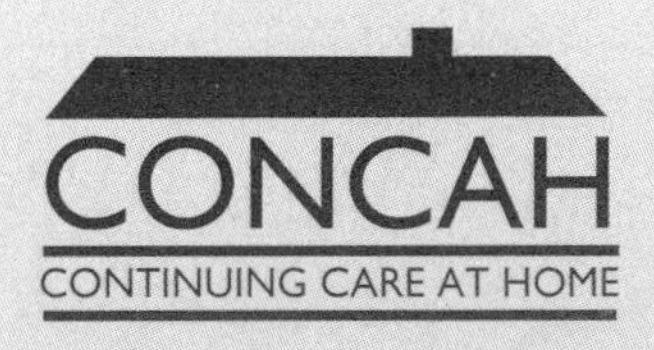

First edition 1996

Published by CONCAH
20 - 25 Glasshouse Yard London EC1A 4JS

British Library Cataloguing in Publication Data. A catalogue record for this book is available from the British Library.

Printed in Great Britain by Norwich Colour Print Ltd,
Unit 2, Drayton Industrial Park, Taverham Road,
Drayton, Norwich NR8 6RL

Design: Rachel Williams Design,
160b Liverpool Road, London N1 1LA

Produced by Jill Fardell Education Publishing Ltd.

ISBN-1-901215-00-8

Acknowledgments

We thank the following people who gave freely of their time to produce this compendium:

AUTHORS

Dr Jim Brockbank (General Practitioner)

Mrs Margaret Buttigieg (health visitor): Regional Nurse Director, S&WRHA, former Director Health Visitor's Association

Ann Crack MSc, MCSP: (community physiotherapist): Richmond, Twickenham and Roehampton Health Care Trust

Professor Pam Enderby (speech and language therapist): Chair of Community Rehabilitation, University of Sheffield

Mrs Angela Hinchcliffe (speech and language therapist): Paraclinical Research Fellow

Dr Bob Jones (General Practitioner(ret)): former Chairman of CONCAH

Dr Sunni Mandana: Consultant Clinical Psychologist, Castle Hill Hospital, Hull

Dr Neil Matson: Chartered Clinical Psychologist, Exeter Community Health Service Trust

Ms Margaret Mattingly (Social worker): Principal Manager, Health and Disability, Royal Borough of Kingston Community Services

Mr Phill Watson: Carers National Association

Mr Brian Roger: Professional Development Officer, Community Psychiatric Nurses' Association

Ms Sue Thomas: Community Adviser, Royal College of Nursing

National Information Forum, for contributions from their *Signposts* book (pub Oct 1996)

INFORMATION AND ADVICE

Royal College of Nursing

Royal College of Speech and Language Therapists

The Chartered Society of Physiotherapy

The College of Occupational Therapists

CRITICAL READER

Dr Chris Clough: Director of Neurosciences, King's College Hospital, London

TESTERS

Our thanks to all the health and social services professionals in the community who tested the compendium. Their time and expertise was invaluable in the development of the book.

STRUCTURAL EDITOR

Lynn Earnshaw: Editorial and Publishing Services.

Contents

and publications it examines the roles and interactions of the different members of the team. It is not possible to put a 'price tag' on caring, and those who have contributed to the work of the organisation and to this compendium have given freely of their time and expertise.

I hope that this compendium will not only help members of the teams who respond so generously to the needs of the disabled, but will also be a beacon illuminating the fact that commitment and compassion are as important as accountability in respecting the intrinsic value of every human being.

Professor David Morrell
OBE, KSG, FRCP, FRCGP, FFPHM

Visiting Professor - General Practice
University of Plymouth

Former President of the BMA

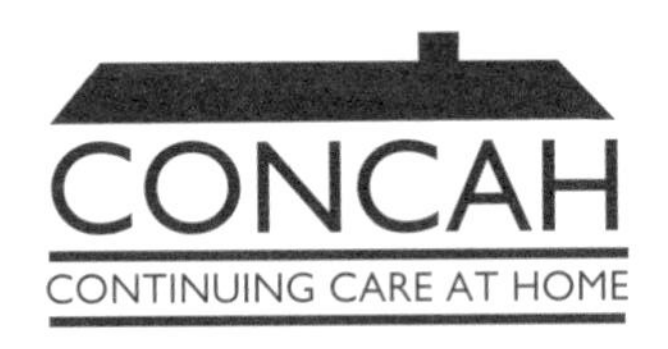

CONCAH, the Continuing Care at Home Association, is a national charity whose members are predominantly nurses, health visitors, general practitioners, therapists, social workers and others who provide primary care.

Formed in 1992, its prime objective is:

'to improve the relief at home of those people living with chronic illness or disability by advancing the learning and understanding of those caring for such people.'

CONCAH's activities include practice workshops, conferences, study days and seminars supported by the production of books, reports and information resources.

DEDICATED TO

Dr Bob Jones
former Chairman and founding member of CONCAH for his vision, commitment and leadership.

1. Introduction

CONCAH aims
'to improve the relief at home of people living with chronic illness or disability by advancing the learning and understanding of those caring for such persons.'

'In 24 per cent of people with disabilities the medical cause is a chronic incurable neurological condition'
Royal College of Physicians, 1986[1].

Doctors and nurses working in primary care can at any time be faced by someone seeking information about an incurable neurological condition which they have never seen before and may never see again in their professional lives. Or someone recently diagnosed may consult them asking to be put in touch with a charity or other voluntary agency which could provide support.

This compendium is designed to provide easy and quick access to relevant and up-to-date information on a comprehensive range of neurological conditions, from the relatively common to the very rare, together with signposts indicating where further support may be obtained.

How to use this compendium

The structure of this book is designed to lead readers in a logical succession - from basic information about neurological conditions, presented in alphabetical order, through to a sixth section providing an up-to-date (1996) list of voluntary agencies who are involved in providing advice and services to people with disability.

Where relevant throughout the book, cross references are made between sections to guide the user to related issues and information. These cross references are signposted by the hand symbol in the left margin.

Cross reference symbol

Section 2: Factfile gives brief, succinct descriptions of the essential features of 24 neurological conditions in a standard factsheet format. These features include:

- The medical aspects of the condition
- The social, psychological and practical issues and problems facing sufferers and their carers
- Important information about what support is available, and where it can be located

Section 3: Some common problems contains summaries and discussion of ten major problem areas experienced by people with incurable neurological conditions, and their domestic carers.

Section 4: Professional roles in continuing care looks at the contributions that can be made by different groups of professionals to the care of disabled people with neurological conditions in the community.

Section 5: Managing continuing care gives an outline of principles appropriate to the ongoing management of people with incurable neurological conditions.

Section 6: Some useful addresses lists the major charities and agencies which provide services and support for people with chronic conditions and disability. This section also contains some blank pages which can be used to compile a directory of local services, which will relate specifically to the needs of your patients, their carers and other members of the primary care team in your area.

CONCAH plans to update this compendium as required, and would welcome comments and suggestions for possible amendments to be incorporated in future editions.

The address is:
CONCAH Compendium
CONCAH Office
20 - 25 Glasshouse Yard
London EC1A 4JS

Reference

1. Royal College of Physicians (1986) Physical Disability in 1986 and beyond: a report of the Royal College of Physicians. *Journal of the Royal College of Physicians,* **20:3,** 160 - 194.

2. *Factfile*

CONTENTS

Alzheimer's disease

FACTFILE 2

VARIATIONS	Senile dementia of Alzheimer's type. Early onset dementia. Pick's disease - progressive dementia in younger people.
PREVALENCE	Alzheimer's disease is the commonest cause of progressive dementia and severe dementia. Approximately 15% of those aged over 65 years of age are demented to a significant degree and 50% of these have Alzheimer's disease. GPs with 10,000 patients can expect to have 100 people with dementia on their lists, 40% of whom will have Alzheimer's disease (Alzheimer's Disease Society figures). It is slightly more common in women. The prevalence of dementia has never been determined but there are thought to be 17,000 people in the UK with early onset dementia.
AGE AT ONSET	Late middle life.
CAUSE	The cause is not yet fully understood. In early onset dementia - the rarer form - there is thought to be a genetic component. Families in which Alzheimer's disease is transmitted through an autosomal dominant gene are fully documented. Senile dementia of Alzheimer's type

is not fully understood. There may be evidence of a genetic component.

Pathology

The brain of a person who dies with advanced Alzheimer's disease is severely atrophied. Many neurones contain neurofibrillary tangles and there are large numbers of amyloid plaques.

Common presentation and symptoms

Intellectual deterioration including: loss of memory (the patients may have some insight into their condition especially in the early stages), depression, disorientation, confusion.

Common major symptoms include:

- Depression
- Loss of short term memory
- Repetitiveness
- Disorientation
- Wandering
- Failure to carry out normal, routine activities of daily living

Prognosis

Progressive, incurable disease with variable speed of development.

Common psychological and emotional problems

Problems, including those listed, are unique to the individual. They do not present in any particular order, and some may not appear at all.

- Loss of ability to perceive, concentrate, orientate
- Loss of ability to remember, learn or reason
- Lack of emotional response and consideration for others
- Depression and/or anxiety

* Delusions
* Fragmented thought processes leading to repetitive, disordered and fragmented speech (dysphasia)

Physical problems usually occur in the later stages. These include:

* Problems with movement and co-ordination
* Weight loss
* Incontinence
* Visuospatial problems - less able to compensate for physical disabilities

Social aspects and problems

Increasing dependency and risk of harm through neglect and isolation.

Family/carers' problems

As the disease progresses, the need for constant supervision and support in daily living can dominate the carer's life.

The need to maintain hygiene, diet, warmth and prevent wandering can be difficult and upsetting.

Increasing responsibility and lack of respite can lead to feelings of grief, anger, guilt, aggression, physical and mental exhaustion.

Roles of professionals

The multidisciplinary team, for example, the general practitioner, community nurses, community psychiatric nurses, clinical psychologists will:

* Assess physical, mental, behavioural and social problems and identify strengths and remaining skills

- Involve the patient and the carer in the assessment process
- Provide explanation and advice
- Identify/manage treatable problems e.g. depression in the early stages and mental disturbance later on
- Identify carer's needs and whether they are being met. Identify appropriate skills and services to meet these needs
- Regularly review the needs of the patient and family carers
- Arrange consistent support for family carers to include financial, domestic and social help, and acceptable respite

INFORMATION AND SUPPORT

Alzheimer's Disease Society
10 Greencoat Place
London SW1P 1PH
Tel: 0171 306 0606
Fax: 0171 306 0808

National office, 13 regional offices, 300+ branches, support groups, carers' contacts.

Services provided:
Information and advice
Respite
Self-help groups
Financial support
Campaigning

Publications include:
Dementia in the Community: Management strategies for General Practice.

Ataxia

Ataxia is a symptom - lack of co-ordinated movement.

VARIATIONS	Hereditary ataxia of unknown cause: Early onset - Friedreich's ataxia is the most common. Late onset - cerebellar ataxia: very rare, autosomal dominant condition (see page 12).
	Hereditary ataxia with metabolic cause - e.g.: Hartnup's disease, Bassen-Kornzweig disease, Batten's disease - see neurological textbooks.
	Ataxia telangiectasia - Louis-Bar syndrome (see page 14).
	FRIEDREICH'S ATAXIA
PREVALENCE	No data. Rarely seen in general practice.
AGE AT ONSET	Mean age: 10 - 12 years.
	Symptoms may present between 4 and 20 years.
CAUSE	Autosomal recessive inheritance.
PATHOLOGY	Sclerosis of the dorsal and lateral columns of the spinal cord.
COMMON PRESENTATION AND SYMPTOMS	Gait slowly becomes more irregular and clumsy: this may be preceded by foot or spinal deformity.
	The child may walk on a broad base and lurch from side to side.

Other symptoms include:

- Clumsiness of fine movement
- Tremor
- Weakness
- Impaired vision and hearing
- Speech difficulties - speech may become unintelligible
- Diabetes in 10% of cases
- Cardiac failure and arrhythmia which are common
- Associated skeletal deformities - especially severe scoliosis - which may require surgery

Prognosis

Progressive disability with mobility, skeletal, cardiac, speech problems.
No cure.
Variable, but for some, death within 20 years of onset.

Common psychological and emotional problems

Depression.
Frustration.
Isolation due to both physical and communication difficulties.

Social aspects and problems

Difficulties accessing education.
Social isolation.

Family/carers' problems

Strain on family and siblings as dependency needs and physical/emotional problems increase.
Other problems include:

- Risk of job loss
- Loss of independence
- Isolation - physical, social and emotional
- Financial difficulties
- Lack of respite facilities/support

Roles of professionals

The provision of physio-, speech and language and occupational therapy services within the community is essential.

Medical care would, when relevant, include: diabetic control, care of cardiac problems, prevention of muscle spasm, surgery for skeletal deformities.

The multidisciplinary team will also continue to provide:

- Medical, social and educational support for the child
- Advice and instructive support for the carers to help minimise their problems

Information and support

Ataxia
Copse Edge
Thursley
Elstead
Godalming
Surrey GU8 6DJ
Tel: 01252 702864
Fax: 01252 703715

National office, local branches and contacts.

Services provided:
Information
Advice
Financial help and support to families and sufferers

Ataxia cerebellar

VARIATIONS	Late onset hereditary ataxia. Autosomal dominant cerebellar ataxia.
PREVALENCE	Very rare.
AGE AT ONSET	Ranges from the third to fifth decade of life or later.
CAUSE	Autosomal dominant inheritance. X-linked inheritance and a sporadic form have been described.
PATHOLOGY	Cerebellar degeneration.
COMMON PRESENTATION AND SYMPTOMS	Clinical manifestations may vary considerably between individuals within families and between families. Symptoms include: • Dysarthria • Intention tremor of the upper limbs • Ataxic gait • Dementia • Optic atrophy • Extrapyramidal rigidity
PROGNOSIS	Variable, slow progression. Wheelchair use likely within 10-20 years.
COMMON PSYCHOLOGICAL AND EMOTIONAL PROBLEMS	Depression, anger, frustration. Physical, emotional and social isolation. Problems resulting from increasing dependency.
SOCIAL ASPECTS AND PROBLEMS	Isolation, job loss, loss of independence, financial problems.

FAMILY/CARERS' PROBLEMS

Strain on family as dependency needs and physical/emotional problems increase. Other problems include:

- Risk of job loss
- Loss of independence
- Isolation - physical, social and emotional
- Financial difficulties
- Lack of respite facilities/support

ROLES OF PROFESSIONALS

Speech and language, occupational and physio-therapy services provided in an integrated manner within the community are essential.

Integrated medical care would include management of depression, incontinence, visual disturbances and intellectual deterioration.

INFORMATION AND SUPPORT

Ataxia
Copse Edge
Thursley
Elstead
Godalming
Surrey
GU8 6DJ
Tel: 01252 702864
Fax: 01252 703715

National office, local branches and contacts.

Services provided
Information
Advice
Financial help and support to families and people with ataxia

FACTFILE 2

Ataxia telangiectasia

SYNONYM	Louis-Bar syndrome.
PREVALENCE	Very rare.
AGE AT ONSET	Usually presents in toddlers. Affected children usually unable to walk by 12 years of age.
CAUSE	Autosomal recessive inheritance.
PATHOLOGY	Progressive cerebellar degeneration accompanied by cutaneous vascular lesions.
COMMON PRESENTATION AND SYMPTOMS	Poor co-ordination; poor speech, eye and hand control. Telangiectasia of conjunctiva (small red spots visible), later evident in the pinnae, face and limb flexures. Immunoglobulin deficiency which may lead to recurrent infections and malignancies.
PROGNOSIS	The disease may be fatal within the second or third decade of life due to the risks of: • Recurrent infection, especially chest infection • High incidence of cancer • Progressive cerebellar degeneration
COMMON PSYCHOLOGICAL AND EMOTIONAL PROBLEMS	Physical, emotional and social isolation resulting from increasing dependency and recurrent infection.
SOCIAL ASPECTS AND PROBLEMS	Need for constant supervision to avoid physical injury.

Social isolation.
Difficulties accessing education.

FAMILY/CARERS' PROBLEMS

Strain on family and siblings as dependency needs and physical/emotional problems increase. Other problems include:

- Risk of job loss
- Loss of independence
- Isolation - physical, social and emotional
- Financial difficulties
- Lack of respite facilities/support

ROLES OF PROFESSIONALS

Speech and language, occupational and physio-therapy services within the community are essential.

Integrated medical care would include management of infection and malignancy if it occurs.

INFORMATION AND SUPPORT

Ataxia Telangiectasia Society
33 Tuffnells Way
Harpenden
Herts AL5 3HA
Tel: 01582 761437

National committee. Work undertaken by various members on a voluntary basis.

Services
Information
Support for families of newly diagnosed patients
Counselling
Family meetings
Special clinic for people with AT
Newsletter

Cerebral palsy

VARIATIONS

Cerebral palsy is a syndrome of muscular weakness resulting from a non-progressive injury to the developing nervous system. It is classified according to the pattern of motor involvement: spastic; dystonic; ataxic and mixed forms. Mixed forms are the commonest.

PREVALENCE

2 per 1000 live born children in most developed countries (ascertained at school entry).

Prevalence of all types of cerebral palsy in babies with a birth weight of 1501 - 2500 grams, is 1 : 100 of neonatal survivors.

AGE AT ONSET

From birth onwards.

CAUSE

It is usually associated with:

- Maternal infections
- Antenatal complications resulting in fetal hypoxia
- Abnormal labour or delivery
- Intra-partum asphyxia - the degree of asphyxia needed to produce brain injury increases as gestational age decreases
- Neonatal illness - particularly neurological
- Meningitis
- Encephalitis
- Trauma including non-accidental injury
- Hypoxia during major operations -

especially major cardiac surgery for severe congenital heart defects

Less frequently, may be due to genetic conditions.

PATHOLOGY

Non-progressive damage to:

- The developing brain
- The brain during or after birth

COMMON PRESENTATION AND SYMPTOMS

Among the first signs are:
- The baby may be floppy, fail to respond or thrive
- Delayed motor development
- Involuntary muscle movement or abnormal gait patterns

Spastic cerebral palsy: muscles are tight, tense and weak.

Dyskinetic cerebral palsy: muscles rapidly change from floppy to tense with involuntary movements. Less control of the tongue and vocal cords causing speech difficulties.

Ataxic diplegia cerebral palsy: clumsiness, lack of balance, poor co-ordination, shaky hand movements and jerky speech.

Delayed motor development. Involuntary muscle movement or abnormal gait patterns.

Any impairment of mental, linguistic, visual, auditory and sensory function needs to be assessed.

Associated handicaps could include: strabismus, refractive errors, deafness, contractures and epilepsy.

Prognosis

It is not possible to predict the degree of motor disability and resulting functional handicaps until the child is at least 5 - 10 years of age as nervous system maturation continues into adolescence.

Improvement often takes years and will be influenced by the level of specialist help and therapy as well as social and environmental factors.

Common psychological and emotional problems

Isolation, depression and frustration.
Communication problems.
Relationship difficulties (including sexual difficulties).

Social aspects and problems

Depends on the nature and degree of the impairment and consequent handicap. The person with cerebral palsy may experience:

- Restricted independence
- Frustration
- Lack of educational, social and employment opportunities
- Financial difficulties in adulthood

Family/carers' problems

Depends on the nature and degree of the impairment and consequent handicap. There may be:

- Strain on family and siblings
- Physical strain from lifting, helping with mobility and other activities
- Loss of independence
- Isolation - physical, social and emotional
- Financial pressures
- Lack of respite facilities and support

Roles of professionals

A multidisciplinary team of speech and language, occupational and physio- therapists and the health visitor would work together to:

- Identify and manage associated handicaps and complications
- Prevent secondary deprivation handicap
- Provide support for families
- Promote independence

Children who have been subjected to the risk factors (described in Cause) but who have no obvious impairment should be assessed at regular intervals.

Information and support

SCOPE
Head Office:
12 Park Crescent
London WIN 4EQ
Tel: 0171 636 5020
Fax: 0171 436 2601

Research Department:
16 Fitzroy Square
London WIP 6LP
Tel: 0171 387 9571
Fax: 0171 388 9775

SOS
(Stars Organisation Supporting action for people with Cerebral Palsy)
Wakes Hall
Wakes Colne
Colchester CO6 2DB
Tel: 01787 222044
Fax: 01787 222649

FACTFILE 2

Charcot Marie Tooth disease

VARIATIONS	Peroneal muscular atrophy. Hereditary motor and sensory neuropathy, types I-IV.
PREVALENCE	Very rare in general practice: less than 1 in 10,000 patients.
AGE AT ONSET	Can present throughout life, but commonly in childhood.
CAUSE	Hereditary: autosomal dominant inheritance; autosomal recessive.
PATHOLOGY	Due to a diffuse degeneration of the myelin sheath or of the axon itself, depending on type.
COMMON PRESENTATION AND SYMPTOMS	Wasting of muscles below the knees. Later weakness and wasting of the small hand muscles. Poor balance. Scoliosis. Bilateral foot drop. Claw and hammer toes. Respiratory problems (occasionally).
PROGNOSIS	Very variable. Slowly progressive symmetrical disorder. Normal life expectancy. Some dependent on a wheelchair after 20 - 30 years. Others are minimally affected, or make do with appropriate orthoses.
COMMON PSYCHOLOGICAL AND EMOTIONAL PROBLEMS	Severe frustration over a long period; physical, emotional and social isolation problems result from increasing dependency.

SOCIAL ASPECTS AND PROBLEMS

Dependent on others for help with activities of daily living such as dressing, bathing, mobility.

Lack of understanding and therefore support from health and social service professionals (due to the rarity of the condition).

FAMILY/CARERS' PROBLEMS

Increasing dependency of the person with the disease creates physical, emotional and social problems for the family carers and other siblings:

- Possible job loss to increase level of care and support
- Loss of independence as the condition progresses
- Physical, social and emotional isolation
- Financial pressures
- Lack of respite facilities and support

ROLES OF PROFESSIONALS

A multidisciplinary team including occupational and physio- therapists and health visitor would work together to manage the physical and psychological problems for the patient and family carers.

There may be a need for orthoses and other appliances. Surgical correction of foot deformity or tendon transfer may be necessary.

INFORMATION AND SUPPORT

Charcot Marie Tooth International
121 Lavernock Road
Penarth
South Glamorgan CF64 3QG
Tel: 01222 709537

National Executive Committee.
Some local groups.

Services

Support

Information

Advice

Annual General Meeting and mini conference

Quarterly newsletter

Creutzfeldt-Jacob disease

FACTFILE 2

VARIATION	New Variant of Creutzfeldt-Jacob disease (NVCJD).
PREVALENCE	CJD occurs worldwide at an annual incidence of about 1: 1 million population. In the UK the provisional figure for 1995 is 43 new cases. NVCJD was described in the UK in March 1996. 11 cases in people under 42 years of age were documented.
AGE AT ONSET	CJD presents in late middle age (average age 63). For the 11 cases of NVCJD documented by March 1996, the average age was 27 years.
CAUSE	The agent is believed to be a protein, the prion protein, which is highly resistant to physical and chemical inactivation. The incubation period is variable, on average between 5 and 15 years. CJD does not behave like a conventional infectious disease, and there is no risk of spread within families. CJD is not transmitted from mother to child in pregnancy or through breast milk. The Department of Health has developed clear guidelines regarding occupational exposure, environmental risks, foodstuffs and

pharmaceutical products, and a directed programme of research and development is currently in progress.

Pathology

A progressive encephalopathy arising from a vacuolar spongiform degeneration of the cerebral cortex. There is no predictive test for classical CJD or for the new variant (NVCJD), and definitive diagnosis can only be made at post-mortem.

Common presentation and symptoms

Non-specific in the early stages. Can include dizziness, fatigue, insomnia, poor concentration, behavioural change and blurred vision.

Focal signs and symptoms can include ataxia, cognitive impairment, aphasia, limb weakness and fits.

In the later stages, weight loss, incontinence, visuospatial problems also occur.

Prognosis

Progressive incurable disease. CJD is usually fatal within 6 months. NVCJD has a tendency to last longer, up to 23 months.

Common psychological and emotional problems

Fatigue, cognitive impairment, problems with movement and co-ordination can all be distressing in the early stages. The onset of dementia is rapid in classical CJD.

Social aspects and problems

Rapid onset of total dependency. Patients are often managed in neurological units or general medical wards.

FAMILY/CARERS' PROBLEMS	Emotional support, information, and practical support in managing symptoms such as incontinence.
ROLES OF PROFESSIONALS	If management at home is to be considered, then the widest spectrum of primary and secondary care involvement will be needed.
	There is no reason for GPs to change their referral patterns to specialists in cases of dementia or ataxia because of NVCJD. All neurologists, including paediatric neurologists, have been advised in detail by the CJD Surveillance Unit which was set up by the Department of Health and the Scottish Home and Health Department in May 1990.
INFORMATION AND SUPPORT	Further information on CJD for health care professionals can be obtained from: Room 510a Skipton House 80 London Road London SE1 6LW
	Information for patients and their family carers is available from The CJD Support Network c/o The Alzheimer's Disease Society 10 Greencoat Place London SW1 1PH Tel: 0171 306 0606 Fax: 0171 306 0808

Dysphasia

VARIATIONS	Dysphasia is a symptom: the difficulty of translating thoughts into language and understanding language. Aphasia is the same condition but suggests a complete loss of language. Many who work with people with dementia would talk of 'language of confusion' not dysphasia.
PREVALENCE	Dysphasia due to stroke - 65 per 10,000 patients. Dysphasia due to other causes - prevalence not known.
AGE AT ONSET	Depends on the cause.
CAUSE	Cerebro-vascular accident - most common cause. Other causes include: head injury, cerebral tumour, raised intracranial pressure and metabolic disorder. Later stages of dementia.
PATHOLOGY	Depends on the cause. The left hemisphere is affected in 99% of right-handed and 60% of left-handed aphasic people.
COMMON PRESENTATION AND SYMPTOMS	Impaired speech and language. Impaired comprehension, expression, reading and writing skills. An 'unseen' disability, the full extent of which is often under-estimated.
PROGNOSIS	Depends on the cause.

Slow improvement possible.
For people who have had a stroke, speech and language therapy may result in continuing improvement even after motor disability has ceased to improve.

COMMON PSYCHOLOGICAL AND EMOTIONAL PROBLEMS	Depression. Frustration. Emotional and therefore social isolation. Disrupted relationships due to communication difficulties. Change of personality (occasionally).
SOCIAL ASPECTS AND PROBLEMS	Isolation. Loss of independence. Loss of job. Financial difficulties.
FAMILY/CARERS' PROBLEMS	Increase in responsibility. Dependency of the person with dysphasia. Possible job loss. Loss of independence. Physical, social and emotional isolation. Financial pressures.
ROLES OF PROFESSIONALS	A multidisciplinary team will assess needs, and provide: • Speech and language therapy • Physio/occupational therapy • Explanation and support for spouse and family • Management of other related conditions (when present) e.g. depression, epilepsy, intracranial

malignancy or other neurological illnesses
- Access to computer aids
- Social service support for carers as well as the person with dysphasia

INFORMATION AND SUPPORT

Action for Dysphasic Adults (ADA)
1 Royal Street
London SE1 7LL
Tel: 0171 261 9572
Fax: 0171 928 9542

National office and local branches. ADA acts as a pressure group through involvement in larger umbrella organisations.

Services
Support
Information
Advice
Annual General Meeting and mini conference
Quarterly newsletter

Dystonia

VARIATIONS	Dystonia is a syndrome - muscular contraction which results in a tendency to maintain a persistent abnormal posture. Focal, segmental, generalised, task specific.
PREVALENCE	Unknown.
AGE AT ONSET	Very variable. Children are particularly affected.
CAUSE	Underlying cause unknown in the majority of cases. History of an illness or injury which has damaged the basal ganglia. Drug induced: Neuroleptic drugs can cause parkinsonism, acute dystonia, akathisia and tardive dyskinesia. Children and young adults are particularly susceptible. The incidence of drug induced dystonia is often dose dependent - approximately 35% for all conditions except acute dystonia where the incidence is 2 - 5%.
PATHOLOGY	The pathogenesis is not clear. Some dystonia patients have illness or injury which damages the basal ganglia.
COMMON PRESENTATION AND SYMPTOMS	Involuntary disabling and extremely painful muscle spasms. Blepharospasm (inability to see for long periods). Writer's cramp (problems with writing and other tasks).

Laryngeal dystonia (inability to speak or make oneself understood).
Spasmodic torticollis - twisting movements of head.

Prognosis

Largely depends on the underlying disorder.

Drug treatment and local botulinum injections can give some symptomatic relief.

Common psychological and emotional problems

Pain, inability to make oneself understood, inability to sit, stand or lie still - all these impact on the psychological and emotional well-being of the person with dystonia.

Children are particularly affected.

Social aspects and problems

Severe handicap and inability to communicate lead to:

- Isolation
- Depression
- Frustration
- Increasing dependency
- Educational difficulties

Family/carers' problems

The person with dystonia may need constant supervision and help.

Children can become severely handicapped leading to:

- Strain on families and other siblings
- Possible job loss
- Loss of independence
- Physical, social and emotional isolation
- Financial pressures

Roles of professionals

The multidisciplinary team would provide:

- Physio/occupational therapy - relaxation exercises
- Speech and language therapy - especially in laryngeal dystonia
- Specialist neurological care and support
- Explanation and support for family
- Social services support for the person with dystonia and the family
- Botulinum service for focal dystonias and blepharospasm

Information and support

The Dystonia Society
Weddel House
13 - 14 West Smithfield
London EC1A 9HY
Tel: 0171 329 0797
Fax: 0171 329 0689

Central office and local branches. Self-help groups and 24 area contacts around the country.

Services
Information for those with dystonia and carers
Information for medical professionals
Dystonia video
Welfare advice and support
Local self-help groups and special literature for children and parents
Promoting research into the cause of dystonia and a possible cure
Newsletter

Epilepsy

VARIATIONS	Epilepsy is repeated seizures of cerebral origin. Variations are: generalised seizures; partial seizures.
PREVALENCE	In children under 16: approximately 7 per 1000. In adults: 1 in 200.
AGE AT ONSET	Can occur at any age. 75% diagnosed under 20 years of age.
CAUSE	Known causes categorised as symptomatic, relate to disturbances within the brain and may be due to: • Head injury • Cerebro-vascular accident • Tumours • Congenital factors - structural abnormalities of the brain; birth asphyxia • Infection, such as meningitis, encephalitis, viral infection, brain abscess Seizures of unknown cause are called idiopathic or cryptogenic.
PATHOLOGY	Seizures are the result of abnormal activity within the brain. The type of seizure depends on the part of the brain which is affected.
COMMON PRESENTATION AND SYMPTOMS	Presentation may be with either generalised or partial seizures. The earliest symptoms may only be discerned by the person involved.

Generalised seizures may present as:

- An absence: the person looks blank and stares for a few seconds, oblivious to external stimuli - carries on activities immediately afterwards, often unaware of what happened. Most common in childhood and adolescence
- Atonic seizure: the body loses all muscle tone and goes floppy
- Tonic seizure: the whole body stiffens as muscles tighten
- Tonic/clonic: the body stiffens; muscles then convulse

Partial seizures may be:

- Simple: slight tingling or twitching in an isolated part of the body; experience strange tastes or smells; no loss of consciousness. This may be the precursor (aura) of other types of seizures
- Complex partial: may include:
  - ~ Impaired consciousness
  - ~ Disorientation
  - ~ Confusion, strange behaviour
  - ~ Strong emotional states
  - ~ Confused meaningless speech
- Secondary generalisation
  - ~ Brain activity is partial initially but then becomes generalised

PROGNOSIS

A good prognosis is associated with a short history, infrequent seizures and a good initial response to treatment. 70% stop having seizures with optimal drug treatment.

Although 50% of treated patients need treatment for more than 5 years, 15 years after initial diagnosis only 30% continue to have seizures.

Common psychological and emotional problems

When the condition is first diagnosed, the person (adults and older children) may experience some or all of the following:

- Shock
- Denial
- Anxiety (which may continue for some time)
- Anger at the impact of the diagnosis on activities, lifestyle and employment prospects

Effects of medication may cause emotional and behavioural changes. Children may become hyperactive.

Social aspects and problems

There is still a stigma attached to epilepsy which is due to a lack of understanding of the condition.

The restrictions which may be imposed by the condition may cause the person with epilepsy to feel different or isolated.

Children may become hyperactive due to the medication, causing problems at school, socially and within the family at home.

Adolescents and adults may be excluded from some activities including:

- Some sports
- Jobs and training
- Driving

UK law stipulates that a driving licence will be issued to people with epilepsy if:

- They have been completely free of seizures for one year; or
- They have had a pattern of seizures which occur only when they are asleep, for the past three years

To hold a PCV (Passenger Carrying Vehicle) or LGV (Large Goods Vehicle) licence a person must have been totally free of seizures and anti-epileptic medication for at least ten years. S/he must also have no neurological evidence of a continuing liability to seizures.

If someone already holds a driving licence when diagnosed with epilepsy, s/he must stop driving and notify the DVLA immediately.

FAMILY/CARERS' PROBLEMS

Coping with the problems experienced by the person with epilepsy:

- Unpredictability of seizures
- Side effects of medication
- Behavioural problems (sometimes)

The distress of seeing a member of the family having a seizure.

In severe cases there may be considerable dependence, with

increasing demands and associated social isolation for the carer.

Roles of professionals

The members of the primary care team would aim to:

- Establish and monitor the correct and rational drug therapy
- Ensure the patient and the carer/s understand the condition and the drugs which are used
- Provide guidance on practical issues such as driving, contraception, planned pregnancy, and measures for emergency treatment of seizures

Consultant neurologists or specialists in epilepsy would be involved in the management of poorly controlled seizures. A patient with socially disabling epilepsy should be referred for consideration of brain surgery.

Nurse specialists would be involved in providing guidance on self-management such as:

- Knowing what triggers seizures and what would help the condition
- Managing stress, sleep and diet

Information and support

British Epilepsy Association
Anstey House
40 Hanover Square
Leeds LS3 1BE
Tel: 0113 243 9393
Fax: 0113 242 8804

Aim is to provide advice to enable people to help themselves.

Central office and local branches.
140 self-help groups.

Services

Information helpline 0800 30 90 30
Internet information services
Literature
Videos
Two conferences per year
Library
Training courses for professionals, people with epilepsy, schools and other members of the public
Membership includes accident insurance

The National Society for Epilepsy

Chalfont St Peter
Bucks SL9 0RJ
Tel: 01494 873991
Fax: 01494 871927

Services

MRI scanning
Medical assessment
Medical research
Rehabilitation
Residential care
Respite care
Videos
Leaflets
Factsheets
Education packages
Advice and information
Conferences
Community network
Associate membership

Guillain-Barré syndrome

VARIATIONS	Guillain-Barré syndrome/polyneuritis - acute idiopathic inflammatory polyneuropathy. Variations include: acute ascending spinal paralysis; acute post infectious polyneuropathy.
PREVALENCE	Very rare in general practice.
AGE AT ONSET	Affects all ages.
CAUSE	No identifiable cause in 50% of cases. Frequently preceded by an enteric or respiratory tract infection 1 - 3 weeks before the onset of symptoms.
PATHOLOGY	An auto-immune response has been postulated - a cell mediated delayed hypersensitivity, in which myelin is stripped off the axons by mononuclear cells. Increase in the protein of the cerebro-spinal fluid without a corresponding increase in cells.
COMMON PRESENTATION AND SYMPTOMS	Neuropathy may commence with severe lumbar or interscapular pain. Paresthesias of the feet – followed by flaccid paralysis and weakness of the legs, ascending to the arms, trunk and face – may be accompanied by a slight fever, bulbar palsy and absent or lessened tendon reflexes. In severe cases the respiratory muscles are affected.

Prognosis	Although most people recover within weeks or months, those more severely affected may have some continuing muscle weakness.
Common psychological and emotional problems	Frustration and chronic fatigue. Problems of adjusting to living with a disability and coping with physical restrictions.
Social aspects and problems	A small number of people may be unable to resume their normal occupation with consequent financial difficulties. Some people with continuing muscle weakness may need aids, support and to have their homes adapted to meet their needs.
Family/carers' problems	Strain on the family of long hospitalisation. Having to live with and adapt to the effects of sudden disability in a member of the family and the consequent change in circumstances for the family as a whole: • Emotional strain • Social pressures • Financial pressures
Roles of professionals	Early referral to a neurologist is essential. A multidisciplinary team will assess needs and provide: • Physiotherapy: this is essential, and hydrotherapy can also be beneficial • Support in helping the patient and

FACTFILE 2

the family to understand and to come to terms with the condition and the physical restrictions it imposes
- Symptom control helped by transcutaneous electrical nerve stimulation (TENS), acupuncture and aromatherapy
- Plasma exchange, a recent development which has been beneficial in more severe cases in the acute stages

INFORMATION AND SUPPORT

Guillain-Barré Syndrome Support Group
Lincolnshire County Council
Council Offices
Eastgate
Sleaford
Lincoln NG34 7EB
Tel: 01529 304615
Fax: 01529 304615

National office
(9.30am - 12.30pm, Mon - Fri)
Volunteers cover at all other times.

Services
Information and advice
Visits
Education of medical professions and public
Local meetings

Huntington's disease

SYNONYMS	Huntington's chorea; chronic (progressive hereditary) chorea; degenerative chorea; hereditary chorea.
PREVALENCE	1: 20,000 Occurs worldwide in all ethnic groups.
AGE AT ONSET	Variable. Generally between ages 30 and 55 years, although in rare cases onset can occur earlier or later in life.
CAUSE	An inherited, autosomal dominant disease. Children of a parent with Huntington's disease have a 1: 2 risk of developing the illness themselves. The risk to their children is 1: 4. It can occur without a previous family history.
PATHOLOGY	The brain is atrophic with conspicuous damage to the cerebral cortex and corpus striatum. Chemical changes such as reduction in various neuro-transmitters which indicate the loss of brain cells.
COMMON PRESENTATION AND SYMPTOMS	Personality change and behavioural problems - 'failure to conform to the norms of socially acceptable behaviour'. Increasingly violent choreiform movements, weight loss,

communication difficulties and dementia.

Prognosis	Death usually follows within 20 years of onset. Life expectancy may be: • Shorter if the onset occurs before 50 years of age • Longer if the onset occurs after 50 years of age
Common psychological and emotional problems	The psychological and emotional problems described under 'Presentation and symptoms'. Depression, especially in coming to terms with the diagnosis and the illness itself. Possible guilt in relation to the genetic risk for existing children.
Social aspects and problems	Loss of independence. Social isolation. Loss of job. Financial difficulties. Lack of understanding of the disease. The social and ethical difficulties associated with predictive genetic testing.
Family/carers' problems	Emotional strain on the family coping with the personality changes and behavioural problems which may result in: • Injury caused by patient's violent movements • Loss of independence • Social isolation

• Financial pressures
• Job loss

ROLES OF PROFESSIONALS

Multidisciplinary care would involve a consultant neurologist; a psychiatrist; speech and language, physio- and occupational therapists who would provide:

• Support and counselling to the patient, carer/family to help them understand and come to terms with the condition and its consequences
• Genetic counselling - the abnormal gene can be identified in all those suffering from the condition, and those who are pre-symptomatic

INFORMATION AND SUPPORT

Huntington's Disease Association
108 Battersea High Street
London SW11 3HP
Tel: 0171 223 7000
Fax: 0171 223 9489

Services
Information
Factsheets
Welfare fund
Regional advisors
Support groups
Local branches

Meningitis

Variations	Bacterial meningitis. Viral meningitis.
Prevalence	Approximately 2000 cases per year of bacterial meningitis notified in England and Wales. Local variations.
Age at onset	Can occur at any age. 70% of cases of bacterial meningitis occur in children.
Cause	Bacterial meningitis: The most common bacteria are meningococcus, pneumococcus and Haemophilus influenzae type B. Viral meningitis: Enteroviruses are responsible for 80 - 90% of diagnosed cases; mumps is responsible for 10 - 20%; herpes zoster, herpes simplex type 2, and measles are less common causes.
Pathology	Infection occurs in the cerebro-spinal fluid within the subarachnoid space and ventricles of the brain and the spinal cord.
Common presentation and symptoms	Bacterial meningitis Early symptoms include: • Malaise • Fever • Headache • Nausea and vomiting • Irritability or drowsiness

Specific, but often late symptoms include:

- Photophobia
- Neck stiffness
- Hamstring spasm - positive Kernig's sign
- Purpuric rash - the absence of a rash does not rule out meningitis

Viral meningitis

Symptoms and signs are similar but in comparison:

- Headache is less severe and tends to be frontal
- Neck stiffness is less marked

Parotid swelling suggestive of mumps, genital vesicles or herpes zoster skin lesions might suggest a specific cause.

PROGNOSIS

Mortality: 5 - 15% with early recognition and appropriate antibiotic treatment.

Viral meningitis is usually self-limiting.

COMMON PSYCHOLOGICAL AND EMOTIONAL PROBLEMS

Problems arising from the residual effects of the meningitis:

- 10% of people recovering from bacterial meningitis have cochlear damage or sensorineural deafness
- 7% may have epilepsy
- Behavioural or learning difficulties
- Neurological deficit and hydrocephalus
- Severe fatigue
- Short term memory loss
- Poor concentration

Social aspects and problems

Children and adults may have problems adapting to the limitations and difficulties imposed by the residual impairments of meningitis.

Children may have particular educational difficulties.

For adults:

- Job loss
- Financial difficulties
- Change in social status

Family/carers' problems

Greater dependency if the patient has significant sequelae such as hearing loss, epilepsy or chronic fatigue.

This may result in:

- Loss of independence
- Social isolation
- Financial pressures
- Job loss

Roles of professionals

It is important for doctors to be aware of the common and major presenting symptoms of meningitis.

Follow - up, support and counselling involving specialists, specialist nurses and appropriate therapists, for the patient and family, particularly when there is residual impairment.

Information and support

The Meningitis Trust
Fern House
Bath Road
Stroud, Glos GL5 3TJ
Tel: 01453 751 738
Fax: 01453 753 588

National office. Network of
voluntary help groups.

Services
Helpline - 0345 538 118
(24 hours - local rates)
Information and advice
Contact with other sufferers/families
Support/counselling
Financial support
Help groups

Motor neurone disease

Variations

Amyotrophic lateral sclerosis (ALS).
Progressive bulbar palsy (PBP).
Progressive spinal muscular atrophy (PMA).

Prevalence

Incidence of 1:100,000 (approximately) - worldwide.
Prevalence of 5:100,000.

In a practice of 10,000, 1 person with MND can be expected. Males more frequently affected - incidence 1.5:1.

Age at onset

Rare under 50 years of age.
Incidence reaches a peak at 70 years of age.

Cause

Unknown.

About 5% of cases are familial, with autosomal dominant inheritance with earlier age of onset.

Pathology

Disease affects the anterior horn cells in the spinal cord, the equivalent cells in the lower cranial nerve nuclei and the neurones of the motor cortex.

The affected cells degenerate.

Common presentation and symptoms

Onset is insidious.
Muscle wasting and weakness (ALS and PMA).
Slurred speech and swallowing difficulties (PBP).
Symptoms may be very slight initially,

but MND can progress rapidly and deterioration can result in:

- Spastic weakness of the legs
- Widespread fasciculation beginning in the shoulder girdle
- Increasing weakness of the limbs leading to severe disability
- Facial weakness
- Respiratory weakness - particularly distressing at night
- Speech becoming unintelligible
- Swallowing difficulties - PBP
- Dementia in rare cases, although intellect is usually unimpaired

Prognosis

Motor neurone disease is an incurable progressive disease. Although the mean time of survival from diagnosis is usually about 3 years, 10% of patients live for more than 10 years with slow onset and progression of disability.

Common psychological and emotional problems

With mental faculties unimpaired, the unrelenting loss of control over environment and physical resources leads to:

- Frustration
- Anger
- Depression
- Grieving

Social aspects and problems

It is vital that the person with MND retains control over his/her life as much as possible and does not become socially isolated or financially dependent.

Family/carers' problems

MND affects the whole family. Grieving begins with the diagnosis. There is frequently a change in roles. The majority of people with MND remain at home so carers face demanding tasks and need support and training in home nursing.

Practical problems arise with the progressive physical losses.

Roles of professionals

The manner in which the diagnosis is given can have a profound effect on psychological adjustment.

It is critical to assure patients that while no cure exists, symptoms can be treated. Patients and carers should be encouraged to seek help and advice.

Community nursing, speech and language, occupational and physiotherapy, are crucial to help maintain a reasonable quality of life.

Effective liaison between the GP, specialists, and members of the multidisciplinary team is vital.

In the later stages of the disease the patient will need:

- Full nursing support
- Aids such as wheelchair, communications systems/equipment
- Percutaneous endoscopic gastrostomy feeding which is being increasingly used
- Counselling for the patient and carers. Carers may, in particular,

need bereavement counselling after the patient dies.

INFORMATION AND SUPPORT

Motor Neurone Disease Association
PO Box 246
Northampton NN1 2PR
Tel: 01604 250505
Fax: 01604 24726

National office; 18 regional staff; 100 local branches.

Services
Helpline for patients and carers: 0345 626262 (local rates)
Information and advice
Support groups
Regional care advisers
Equipment provision
Limited financial assistance

FA

Multiple sclerosis

SYNONYM	Disseminated sclerosis.
PREVALENCE	Global regions of low, medium and high prevalence can be identified: Low - < 5:100,000. Medium - 30:100,000. High - 300:100,000. UK prevalence is approximately 60:100,000. Prevalence is high in Scotland, the highest having been recorded in Shetland and Orkney.
	Annual incidence shows similar variation from 0.4 per 100,000 in South Africa to 9.5 per 100,000 in Orkney.
	Female preponderance is 3:2.
	A general practice of 10,000 patients would expect to have 10 patients with multiple sclerosis.
AGE AT ONSET	Onset is rare in the first decade of life. Steep rise in incidence in the second decade, peaking around 30 years of age and then declining. Onset in people over 50 years is increasingly rare.
CAUSE	Unknown.
	Susceptibility is influenced by genetic factors. The risk in siblings is 1:20 and 1:4 in identical twins.

There appears to be an interplay between individual susceptibility and environmental triggers, the likeliest of which may be a virus or group of viruses.

Ignorance of the etiology of the disease, the immediate causes of relapses and the mechanism of remission has effectively prevented any rational approach to treatment.

PATHOLOGY

The disease inflames the myelin sheath and may lead to permanent scarring of the sheath and secondary damage to the axon.

COMMON PRESENTATION AND SYMPTOMS

The most common symptoms are:

- Blurred or double vision which can persist for a week or more
- Vertigo
- Fatigue
- Weakness of one or more limbs - common onset - dragging of one leg at first after prolonged activity, later obvious during ordinary activity
- Numbness in the limbs - beginning in the feet, spreading in a few days to the waist
- Lack of balance
- Poor mobility
- Incontinence
- Emotional and cognitive problems

PROGNOSIS

Prognosis is variable.

Although incurable with a reduced life expectancy, outcome ranges from:

- Fast-track: 5% of patients who die within 5 years; to

- Benign: 15% of patients who exhibit no significant disability 25 years after onset

COMMON PSYCHOLOGICAL AND EMOTIONAL PROBLEMS	Stress in family relationships. Depression. Frustration due to: • The lack of a rational approach to treatment • The unpredictability of the disease • Loss of independence and the impact on the ability to work Some people may have an early loss of mental acuity.
SOCIAL ASPECTS AND PROBLEMS	Lack of understanding within society of the problems encountered by people living with disability. A variable response from employers and health care professionals. Financial difficulties. Loss of independence. Lack of emotional support. Social isolation.
FAMILY/CARERS' PROBLEMS	Difficulty in obtaining emotional support and practical help, e.g.: • Respite breaks • Financial help • Support in coping with the unpredictability of the disease
ROLES OF PROFESSIONALS	An informed approach from the primary care team to provide appropriate levels of care and support: • Physiotherapy, to improve the ability to walk, and management of

spasticity/contractures

- Occupational therapy and provision of special aids to help in activities of daily living
- Counselling and support for both patient and carer
- Referral to a urologist/continence adviser to advise and assist with continence problems
- Pregnancy counselling - pregnancy does not affect the overall outcome of MS but the risk of relapse increases from 6:1 to 4:1
- District nurses to monitor skin sores
- Social services: respite services, financial advice and help
- Specialist assessments of disability especially spasticity and contractures

INFORMATION AND SUPPORT

The Multiple Sclerosis Society
25 Effie Road
Fulham
London SW6 1EE
Tel: 0171 736 6267
Fax: 0171 736 9861

National office; 18 regional staff; 100 local branches.

Muscular dystrophy

VARIATIONS	The muscular dystrophies are a group of conditions in which progressive degeneration occurs in groups of muscles without abnormality of their innervation. Variations include: Duchenne's muscular dystrophy, Becker's muscular dystrophy, limb-girdle dystrophy, myotonic dystrophy (the most common type).
PREVALENCE	The muscular dystrophies are comparatively rare. Estimated number of cases of all types at any one time in the UK: 5000 - 6000. Duchenne's muscular dystrophy is the most well-known, with an incidence of 13 - 33: 100,000 live male births. A general practice of 10,000 people would expect to have one patient with muscular dystrophy. Predominantly affects males.
AGE AT ONSET	Varies from birth to middle age. Myotonic dystrophy can remain unrecognised. Duchenne's muscular dystrophy is usually recognised within the first 3 years of life.
CAUSE	All forms are genetically inherited: X-linked trait.The exact cause of the muscle wasting is unknown.
PATHOLOGY	Degenerative myopathy.

Etiology may prove to be different in each type of the disease.

Duchenne's muscular dystrophy

Common presentation and symptoms	There is usually weakness and wasting of the muscles of the pelvic girdle which presents as difficulty in walking, climbing stairs, inability to run and frequent falling. Eventually all voluntary muscles may be affected.
Prognosis	Increasing muscular weakness, often progressing rapidly between the ages of 8 - 12 years. Contractures in the later stages. Most affected boys die before they reach 20 years of age usually due to respiratory weakness or heart failure.
Common psychological and emotional problems	Depression and frustration at the progressive nature of the condition and its variability.
Social aspects and problems	Loss of independence. Isolation. Providing care at home is very difficult.
Family/carers' problems	Increasing dependency in an adolescent boy creates heavy physical, emotional and social demands on the carer/family. Difficulties in obtaining practical and emotional support and respite. Job/career loss for the carers.

ROLES OF PROFESSIONALS

The primary care team will aim to provide consistent support for the patient and carers in delaying or alleviating the symptoms:

- Antibiotics for complications such as respiratory and urinary infections
- Physiotherapy to delay the progressive weakness and the onset of contractures; light spinal support to help delay development of skeletal deformity

Physiotherapy and occupational therapy are crucial.

Orthopaedic specialist involvement: surgery may be necessary to control scoliosis or alleviate contractures.

Neurologist: to advise on appropriate management.

INFORMATION AND SUPPORT

Muscular Dystrophy Group of Great Britain & Northern Ireland
7 - 11 Prescott Place
London SW4 6BS
Tel: 0171 720 8055

National charity funding research into treatments and cures for muscular dystrophy and allied muscle wasting conditions. National office and local groups.

Services

Advice and support through Family Care Offices
A national occupational therapist
Grants - the Joseph Patrick Memorial Trust

Myalgic encephalomyelitis (ME)

VARIATIONS	Chronic fatigue syndrome (CFS). Post-viral fatigue syndrome (PVFS).
PREVALENCE	Chronic fatigue is relatively common. Chronic fatigue syndrome: 1% of the population. Myalgic encephalomyelitis: 1- 2:1000. Affects all socio-economic groups.
AGE AT ONSET	Any age including children. Peak incidence is 20 - 40 years of age.
CAUSE	Not fully understood. Entero-viruses, especially coxsackie, herpes and retroviruses may be involved. Depression has been postulated as an etiological factor in at least 50% of patients.
PATHOLOGY	Both immunodepression and activation of the immune system although non-specific, have been described, but no specific pathology has been consistently identified. It is thought there may be a subset of patients in whom abnormality of muscle function may be present.
COMMON PRESENTATION AND SYMPTOMS	Onset may be sudden with no apparent cause, e.g. sudden vertigo. There may be a history of infection of the upper respiratory tract or gastro-intestinal tract. Some cases have a low grade pyrexia usually subsiding within a week.

Subsequent persistent and profound fatigue, both physical and mental, with prolonged recovery time, even after trivial activity.

Symptoms may fluctuate daily or within the day and include:

- Headache
- Giddiness
- Blurred vision
- Muscle tenderness and weakness
- Paresthesia
- Frequency of micturition
- Hyperacusis
- Tinnitus
- Emotional lability
- Impaired tolerance of alcohol
- Circulatory impairment with cold extremities, hyper-sensitivity to climatic change

PROGNOSIS

Approximately one third of people make a complete recovery. One third follow a variable course with fluctuating energy levels less than 50% of normal. One third have severe disability with established chronic symptoms.

COMMON PSYCHOLOGICAL AND EMOTIONAL PROBLEMS

Living within the restrictions of fatigue which, for some, involves inactivity and dependence on others.
Coping with the necessary adjustment to lifestyle.
Loss of confidence.
Emotional lability.
Coping with cognitive impairment.
Frustration and anger.

Social aspects and problems	Lack of understanding of the illness among friends, professionals, colleagues and employers. Incomplete diagnosis. Risk of job loss. Loss of role, finances and independence.
Family/carers' Problems	Understanding the illness and its effects. Dealing with scepticism and disbelief from health care professionals. Obtaining appropriate patient support from health and social services including respite provision. Loss of job or career if the patient becomes increasingly dependent. Coping with the cognitive impairment of the person with ME which can include irritability and mood swings.
Roles of professionals	A team approach is ideal, and good communication between the professionals involved is vital. Acknowledging a real problem exists, obtaining as specific a diagnosis as possible. Providing information to enable the person to: • Understand the illness • Make informed decisions • Acknowledge change • Continue activity • Reorganise his/her life • Deal with unavoidable stress

Drug treatment is aimed at relieving symptoms:

- Sensitivity to drugs is common
- Treatment should begin with smaller doses than normal
- Antidepressants can be helpful for some people
- Those who are not overtly depressed may also benefit from a trial of antidepressants

Simple supportive counselling, coping techniques, cognitive behavioural therapy may help.

Good nutrition is important.

Complementary therapy such as homeopathy or acupuncture can improve relaxation, help in pain control and reduce stress.

Health care professionals should be aware of factors that can cause a relapse or exacerbate symptoms. These include: excess activity, alcohol, intercurrent infection, immunisation, psycho-social stress, surgery or trauma and anaesthetics.

INFORMATION AND SUPPORT

ME Association
Stanhope House
High Street
Stanford le Hope
Essex SS17 0HA
Tel: 01375 642466
Fax: 01375 360256

West Care
White Ladies Road
Clifton
Bristol BS8 2RF
Tel: 0117 9239341

West Care holds a specialist medical reference library and a detailed report on chronic fatigue syndromes supported by the Department of Health which is available for £6.95.

National ME Centre and Centre for ME Syndromes
Disablement Services Centre
Harold Wood Hospital
Romford
Essex RM3 9AR
Tel: 01708 378050
Fax: 01708 378032

Action for ME
PO Box 1302
Wells
Somerset BA5 2WE
Tel: 01749 670799

Myasthenia gravis

Prevalence	Unknown. Occurs in women twice as often as in men. Affects all races. Rarely seen in general practice.
Age at onset	Most commonly begins in early adult life. May also develop in childhood, or as late as the 9th decade.
Cause	It is an auto-immune disorder and closely related to thyrotoxicosis. There are occasionally related associations with diabetes mellitus, rheumatoid arthritis and systemic lupus erythematosus.
Pathology	A disorder of neuromuscular function due to an accumulation of antibodies to acetylcholine receptors at the neuromuscular junction.
Common presentation and symptoms	Abnormal muscle fatigue and exhaustion which may be restricted to a group of muscles or become generalised. It may affect any muscle of the body but especially those of the eye, face, lips, throat, tongue and neck. Ptosis of one or both upper eyelids develops gradually. It is often the first symptom and may soon be associated with double vision.

Difficulty in swallowing or chewing with a deterioration in speech may also be a presenting symptom.

In some cases there is ventilatory insufficiency.

Spontaneous remission can occur which is sometimes complete and long lasting. More often remission is temporary lasting a few months or years, followed by a relapse.

PROGNOSIS	After 10 years or so, many patients enter a static phase with only a moderate response to treatment and a varying degree of residual disability. In rare cases the condition is fatal in the first 2 - 3 years.
COMMON PSYCHOLOGICAL AND EMOTIONAL PROBLEMS	Depression, frustration, isolation due to lack of information and awareness of the condition.
SOCIAL ASPECTS AND PROBLEMS	Poor morale because of the lack of general understanding of the condition and the difficulties it can present. There may be a risk of job loss or loss of independence depending on the variability of relapse and residual disability.
FAMILY/CARERS' PROBLEMS	Problems associated with: • Obtaining patient support • Respite provision • Threat of job loss • Coping with the variability of the condition and disability

Roles of professionals

Skilled neurological review is important.

The primary health care team can provide:

- Education and support for the patient and carer
- Regular assessment and review of patient's and carer's needs
- Specific therapy according to the type and degree of impairment - speech and language, occupational and physio- therapy

Information and support

Myasthenia Gravis Association
Keynesa House
77 Nottingham Road
Derby DE1 3QS
Tel: 01332 290219
Fax: 01332 293641

National office, local branches, regional organisers (paid), regional counsellors (voluntary). Research funding.

Services
Information
Counselling - MGA provides a counselling service of especial help to those who are newly diagnosed

Neurofibromatosis

Synonyms	Von Recklinghausen's disease. Multiple neuroma. Neuromatosis.
Prevalence	Rare - numbers unknown.
Age at onset	Peripheral form (Nf1) can present from birth onwards. Central form (Nf2) is latent and may not present until late teens.
Cause	Inherited autosomal dominant trait. Tends to be more severe when transmitted by a male.
Pathology	Developmental changes in the nervous system, muscle, bones and skin.
Common presentation and symptoms	Peripheral form (Nf1): Café-au-lait spots, axillary or inguinal freckling and neurofibromas on peripheral nerves and spinal roots. There is a 5% risk of malignancy in the neurofibromas and a slight risk of epilepsy. Central form (Nf2): Cranial nerve tumours such as bilateral acoustic neuromas, mental retardation and a tendency to develop gliomas and meningiomas.
Prognosis	Most people with this condition will live a normal life with few medical problems. One third will have complications. In

one third of these people the complications will be serious and possibly life threatening.

Common psychological and emotional problems

The diagnosis can be a shock and cause great anxiety to the patient. They may have difficulty adjusting if they have:

- Disfiguring lesions
- Malignancies
- Epilepsy

Social aspects and problems

People with this condition often feel alone and isolated.
There may be problems in making social adjustments if they have disfiguring lesions or epilepsy.

Family/carers' problems

Parents may have strong feelings of guilt.
Siblings may resent the child with the condition.
Parents will want to know about the disease, its progress and prognosis.
The information available may vary.

Roles of professionals

The primary care team can foster a realistic but positive approach through:

- Information
- Counselling
- Support

Specialist help may be necessary, e.g.:

- Genetic counselling
- Neurosurgical
- Orthopaedic
- Ear, nose and throat

An annual hearing check should be carried out.

CT or MRI scans may be necessary in some cases.

INFORMATION AND SUPPORT

The Neurofibromatosis Association
Head Office
82 London Road
Kingston-upon-Thames
Surrey
BT61 3HP
Tel: 0181 547 1636

FACTFILE 2

Parkinson's disease

PREVALENCE	1:1000 in the UK. Rises after the age of 50 years to 1: 200 at 70 years. Occurs worldwide in all ethnic groups. Slightly more common in men than in women. A general practice of 10,000 could expect to have 11 people with the disease.
AGE AT ONSET	Onset under 40 years is rare. Mean age - 55 years. Thereafter the incidence rises exponentially with increasing age.
CAUSE	Unknown. Research suggests that some people may inherit a genetic susceptibility which, combined with other factors (e.g. environmental), may make them more likely to develop the disease.
PATHOLOGY	Deficiency of dopamine which is produced in the substantia nigra of the basal ganglia, the part of the brain which controls movement. Degeneration of brain stem pigmented nuclei is the crucial feature.
COMMON PRESENTATION AND SYMPTOMS	Onset is insidious. In 70% of people the disease presents as a unilateral tremor. The three cardinal signs of Parkinson's disease are:

- Tremor - which is present at rest, decreased by activity, increases with emotional stress and disappears during sleep
- Rigidity - the result of sustained increase in muscle contraction; may cause muscle pain and stiffness; may be intermittent (cogwheel) or sustained (lead pipe)
- Akinesia - results in slowness of movement, stooped posture, mask-like face, drooling of saliva and shuffling gait

Other signs may include: tiredness, depression, speech problems, swallowing difficulty and constipation.

Most people have normal intellectual and cognitive function.
Up to 20% may develop dementia in the later stages.

PROGNOSIS

10% deteriorate rapidly.
30% deteriorate moderately slowly.
The majority deteriorate very slowly. People in this group can expect to be independent or moderately independent for 10 years or more after diagnosis.

Prognosis will depend on the response to levodopa drugs. It is much worse if there is little response.

COMMON PSYCHOLOGICAL AND EMOTIONAL PROBLEMS

Depression, anxiety and stress occur in the early and later stages and impact on every aspect of life. This may be caused by a combination of the strain of living with the condition and the biochemical changes in the brain.

Many people complain of slowness of thought and defects of memory.

The commonest mental consequence of drug therapy is hallucinosis, but other behaviour disturbances such as schizophreniform psychosis can occur.

20% develop dementia.

SOCIAL ASPECTS AND PROBLEMS

Difficulty in performing activities of daily living such as dressing, toiletting, eating.

Communication difficulties coupled with loss of facial expression and body language impact on social interaction. This can lead to loss of self-esteem and social isolation.

30% of people become clinically depressed.

Drug therapy can have distressing side effects such as rapid swings from mobility to immobility, often several times a day.

Incontinence can be a problem for some in the later stages.

FAMILY/CARERS' PROBLEMS

Because of the long term nature of Parkinson's disease and the fact that it predominantly affects the older population, the family carers themselves are often older people with a disability or poor health.

The needs of the person with the disease and the family carer/s will change over time and dependency often increases. Every person and family carer has different needs, but most require:

- Information
- Respite
- Emotional support
- Financial and practical advice and support

ROLES OF PROFESSIONALS

A multidisciplinary approach is essential; access to a key worker or specialist nurse who will be responsible for ensuring that the needs of the person with Parkinson's disease and the family carer/s are met is often helpful.

Regular assessment is essential as needs change.

Referral to a neurologist or geriatrician with a special interest in Parkinson's disease is important.

Early intervention by the speech and language, physio- and occupational therapists is necessary to maintain the individual's skills and abilities.

Drug treatment needs to be tailored to suit the individual's needs in terms of timing and dosage. Where necessary, specialist advice should be sought.

INFORMATION AND SUPPORT

The Parkinson's Disease Society
22 Upper Woburn Place
London WC1H 0RA
Tel: 0171 383 3513
Fax: 0171 388 5754
Helpline: 0171 388 5759

National office in London, an office in Scotland, 14 field staff, more than 200 local branches, a special section called YAPP&RS for younger people (those of working age) with Parkinson's disease and their families.

Services

Information and advice
Support groups
Publications and videos for professionals and those with, or caring for, someone with Parkinson's disease
Training for professionals and voluntary workers
Promote and fund research (both medical and welfare)
Holidays
Fundraising

Progressive supranuclear palsy

SYNONYM	Steele Richardson Olszewski syndrome.
PREVALENCE	Rare.
AGE AT ONSET	Usually in the 5 - 7th decades. Males are affected more than females. No familial tendency.
CAUSE	Unknown.
PATHOLOGY	Progressive neuro-degenerative disease. Widespread neuronal loss and gliosis in the brain stem.
COMMON PRESENTATION AND SYMPTOMS	Often confused with parkinsonism. Progressive loss of balance (falling backwards). Impaired vision, especially upward and downward gaze. Loss of mobility within 4 years of diagnosis - become wheelchair bound. Dysarthria, swallowing difficulties, dystonic postures and other abnormal movements including tremor, akinesia and rigidity. Mental function may appear impaired due to difficulties in formulating answers.
PROGNOSIS	A progressive disorder which starts insidiously.

Death usually occurs within six years of diagnosis.

Common psychological and emotional problems

Emotional lability, stress, depression and impaired mental function.

Social aspects and problems

A great deal of stress is created as a result of:

- The difficulty in diagnosing the condition which is often mistaken for Parkinson's disease
- Fear of the progression of the disease
- Lack of treatment options

Family/carers' problems

Increasing dependency creates physical, emotional and social strain.

Carers suffer as a result of demands on their time, lack of sleep, respite and practical and emotional support.

Roles of professionals

The carer needs to be well supported from the early stages.

Speech and language, physio- and occupational therapists will be needed to provide advice and to develop strategies to help with speech, swallowing and falling.

In the later stages, full nursing support, wheelchair, communication systems and equipment will be necessary.

In some cases a gastrostomy may be needed.

INFORMATION AND SUPPORT

The Progressive Supranuclear Palsy
(PSP Europe) Association
The Old Factory
Wappenham
nr Towcester
Northamptonshire NN12 8SQ
Tel: 01327 860342
Fax: 01327 860242

National office, local support groups currently in Liverpool, Northern Ireland, Bromley and Sussex.

Services
Information and advice
Support for local PSP groups
Promote research
Raise awareness among professional bodies

FACTFILE 2

Rett syndrome

SYNONYM	Cerebroatrophic hyperammonemia.
PREVALENCE	Occurs exclusively in females. Although rare, the syndrome is the most common cause of profound mental and physical disability in females aged 1 - 10 years.
AGE AT ONSET	Present from birth.
CAUSE	Unknown. Suspected genetic mutation on the X-chromosome.
PATHOLOGY	Cerebral atrophy, mild hyperammonemia and decreased levels of biogenic amines.
COMMON PRESENTATION AND SYMPTOMS	Presents with loss of speech. Progresses slowly and inexorably through childhood to profound mental and physical disability characterised by: • Autistic behaviour • Loss of purposeful use of the hands • Seizures • Dementia • Scoliosis • Loss of independent mobility
PROGNOSIS	Profound physical and mental disability usually occurs when the person is in her 40s.

COMMON PSYCHOLOGICAL AND EMOTIONAL PROBLEMS	Profound mental disability - mental age does not exceed 18 months.
SOCIAL ASPECTS AND PROBLEMS	Total dependency.
FAMILY/CARERS' PROBLEMS	The burden of care can be overwhelming especially as the person ages. Strain on family including siblings as dependency needs and physical/emotional problems increase. Problems include: • Risk of job loss • Loss of independence • Isolation - physical, social and emotional • Financial difficulties • Lack of respite facilities • Lack of support
ROLES OF PROFESSIONALS	Many of the drugs used in other disabling conditions have a place in the management of Rett syndrome. Complicating conditions such as seizures will need to be managed. Speech and language, physio- and occupational therapists will be involved in care, providing for example: • Physiotherapy, hydrotherapy and underwater jet massage which can be helpful • Equipment and aids such as braces,

splints and individualised wheelchairs

Carers will need respite, emotional and practical advice and support.

INFORMATION AND SUPPORT

UK Rett Syndrome Association
29 Carlton Road
London N11 3EX
Tel: 0181 361 5161

National office, local support groups/contacts.

Services

Self-help groups for carers
Information and advice
Advocacy
Diagnostic and therapy clinics
Promote awareness
Encourage best known practice in treatment and care
Annual conference
Support for research

Stroke

VARIATIONS	Cerebro-vascular accident, cerebral infarction. Transient ischaemic attacks (TIAs) - strokes which last less than 24 hours.
PREVALENCE	Every year, about 100,000 people in the UK have their first stroke. A general practice with a population of 10,000 would expect 65 people with a diagnosis of stroke. In North America and Europe the incidence is 1 - 2:1000 population. In developed countries it is the third commonest cause of death after heart disease and cancer. The incidence of transient ischaemic attack (TIA) is unknown.
AGE AT ONSET	Rare under 55 years of age: 90% are aged over 60 years at onset. Stroke can occur in the last trimester of pregnancy or in the puerperium but is very rare (5:10,000 deliveries in the UK).
CAUSE	Risk factors: • Hypertension – the most important • Heart disease of any kind • Peripheral vascular disease • Diabetes mellitus • Cigarette smoking • Obesity • Excess alcohol consumption

- Hyperlipidemia
- The contraceptive pill – the risk of stroke is increased three times and is compounded by smoking and obesity

PATHOLOGY

A stroke is a rapidly developing episode of focal and, at times, global loss of cerebral function due to cerebral infarction, intracerebral haemorrhage or subarachnoid haemorrhage.

Transient ischaemic attack: this is an acute loss of focal, cerebral or ocular function which is presumed to be due to embolic or thrombotic vascular disease, and lasts less than 24 hours.

COMMON PRESENTATION AND SYMPTOMS

Vary according to the location, extent and cause of the lesion. Sudden or relatively sudden (0 - 24 hours) onset of:

- Muscular paralysis - often unilateral
- Sensory loss
- Loss of vision
- Loss of ability to speak
- Unconsciousness

PROGNOSIS

Approximately 25% of people who have a stroke die within 24 hours. A further 25% die within one month.

Of the survivors, half eventually have slight or no disability whereas half remain severely disabled.

Prediction of the probability of survival is unwise during the first week after a stroke. Some patients with apparently severe strokes can recover rapidly.

COMMON PSYCHOLOGICAL AND EMOTIONAL PROBLEMS	Misery, anxiety, frustration and clinical depression are common. Emotional lability may result in spontaneous episodes of crying.
SOCIAL ASPECTS AND PROBLEMS	Loss of mobility and ability to communicate lead to isolation and heavy responsibility for family and carers. Inability to carry out normal activities of daily living increases dependency. The costs of caring for a person at home. Dependency and communication problems can lead to social isolation.
FAMILY/CARERS' PROBLEMS	For family and carers involved with people who eventually have little or no disability, anxiety, fear of recurrence and emotional disturbance may persist. Those who remain severely disabled may create a heavy burden for their carers. The day to day tasks for which they are responsible are often physically demanding, and coping with this dependency has emotional, psychological and social implications. Respite in a form acceptable to patient and carer may be very difficult to achieve.

Roles of professionals

For those who survive a stroke but remain severely disabled, it is likely that they and their family carers will have multiple needs which span professional boundaries.

In order to co-ordinate an effective programme, without duplication or gaps, nurses, physiotherapists, occupational therapists, speech and language therapists, social workers and volunteer support groups should be involved in the care and support of the person with the stroke and the family carer/s.

Information and support

The Stroke Association
CHSA House
Whitecross Street
London EC1Y 8JJ
Tel: 0171 490 7999
Fax: 0171 490 2686

Regional managers, community services.

Services
Information
Telephone advisory service
Information centres
Community services
Welfare grants
Research grants

Tuberous sclerosis

SYNONYM	Bourneville's disease.
PREVALENCE	Rare.
AGE AT ONSET	Birth onwards - seizures are common in infancy.
CAUSE	Inherited, usually autosomal dominant, but sporadic cases can occur. Two genes, one each on chromosomes 9 and 16, are thought to be responsible.
PATHOLOGY	Hamartomatous proliferation of various tissues. High incidence of renal disorder, cerebral astrocytomas and pulmonary disease.
COMMON PRESENTATION AND SYMPTOMS	The most frequent major problems include: • Seizures: 80% • Learning difficulties: 50% • Autism and hyperactivity • Renal disorders • Pulmonary disease • Facial angiofibroma • Acne-like facial rash
PROGNOSIS	30% of those with the condition die by 30 years of age. A proportion stabilise, but many have increasing intellectual problems, resistant epilepsy, or require treatment for brain tumour.

COMMON PSYCHOLOGICAL AND EMOTIONAL PROBLEMS	Autism and attention deficits. Learning difficulties.
SOCIAL ASPECTS AND PROBLEMS	Autistic behaviour, learning difficulties and seizures can lead to depression and social isolation especially in young adults. It may be difficult to find up-to-date information about the condition or doctors who know about it.
FAMILY/CARERS' PROBLEMS	Problems for carers include: • Lack of information • Coping with seizures, learning difficulties, behavioural problems • Sleepless nights • Lack of respite • Job loss • Social isolation
ROLES OF PROFESSIONALS	Autism or behavioural difficulties should be managed appropriately with the help of social services and nurses trained in caring for people with learning difficulties. Social services can assist with placement in special schools which can be beneficial for the person with the condition and the family. Monitoring and treatment of seizures, with ultrasound scan of kidneys, CT or MRI scans of the brain to identify any tumours. Genetic advice for parents and siblings.

Respite for the family carer/s.

Advice and support for the carer/s.

Social services support for the whole family is important.

INFORMATION AND SUPPORT

Tuberous Sclerosis Association
Little Barnsley Farm
Catshill
Bromsgrove
Worcs B61 0NQ
Tel: 01527 871898

Three employed staff members and a network of regional representatives for local support.

Services

Information - a wide range of leaflets is available
Specialist TS clinics
Family Care Officer to visit and advise
Benevolent fund
Meetings for members
Professional study days across the country
International research symposia
Holidays/weekend breaks for mildly affected adults

3. Common problems

Contents

Communication

Communication difficulties which arise as a result of neurological conditions can significantly disable those who live with these conditions.

TYPES OF DISORDER

Dysphasia or aphasia is caused by neurological damage to the dominant cerebral hemisphere, most typically in stroke, but it can also occur as a result of head injury, neurosurgery or cerebral tumour.

It affects the ability to:

- Understand language
- Produce speech and language: for example, to find the correct word, or order words in a sentence (expressive dysphasia)
- Read and write

The extent of dysphasia can range from no speech but good comprehension to fluent speech but severely reduced comprehension, depending on the site of the lesion (Broca's versus Wernicke's aphasia).

People who have experienced dysphasia have likened it to suddenly finding themselves in a land where they do not speak or understand the language. This is a most frightening experience.

Dysarthria or anarthria is an acquired neuromuscular disorder which may result from a stroke in the non-dominant hemisphere of the brain, a number of small strokes or a brain stem lesion. It also occurs in progressive neurological disorders such as Parkinson's disease, motor neurone disease and multiple sclerosis.

Dysarthria affects the ability to produce speech at some stage of the speech chain, for example:

breathing, phonation, co-ordination of breath and voice, resonance or articulation.

People with this condition are able to understand language and to structure their own language, but their speech is typically slurred and unclear. Since their ability to understand and to structure language is unaffected, it may be possible to use alternative methods of communication such as writing, communication aids and computers.

Dyspraxia or apraxia is a motor problem which often accompanies and complicates dysphasia, for example in stroke.

People with this condition are not paralysed, but suffer with involuntary movements which have no purpose. For example, they are able automatically to carry out the oral movements necessary for eating but cannot apply those movements voluntarily in order to produce speech sounds.

Language and dementia. Communication problems in people with dementia are different from those described above:

- **The language problems which develop in dementia are due to difficulties in the use and appropriateness of language rather than the structure and articulation of language.**
- **Unlike dysphasia, the onset of language problems in dementia is gradual and accompanied by other cognitive problems, such as memory loss and confusion.**

This is because they are not caused by problems with the language areas of the brain, but arise as a result of cognitive decline.

Combinations of disorders

People with communication problems often have elements of more than one of the disorders described above. For example, people who have had a stroke often have features of both dysarthria and dysphasia; people with dementia may develop specific dysphasic problems as a result of focal damage; in the latter stages of Parkinson's disease, it is not uncommon to develop some features of confusion which may complicate a diagnosis of dysarthria.

Effects of communication difficulties

Speech and language difficulties remain an 'unseen' disability and it is easy to underestimate the devastating effect they can create.

- Our entire social and working lives are largely directed by our ability to communicate and interact. When a person loses that ability, life becomes completely disrupted, both for the individual and for all those involved with that person.
- We use language not just to communicate with those around us, but to express our individuality and personality. Losing this ability as part of a communication problem often has more far reaching effects than may be apparent at first sight. People often feel disempowered by their communication difficulties and they may feel a loss of identity, personality and status.

In working with people with communication problems, health care professionals need to be aware of the dangers of making assumptions and swift judgements about the severity of the problem in relation to the disability that will face them. For example:

- A mild dysarthria may represent a massive loss for someone who is used to public speaking and whose livelihood depends on that ability, whereas it might be less of a problem for someone whose work did not require this level of communication skills.
- A person who has recovered well from an expressive dysphasia may be judged to have done extremely well, and yet the mildest of residual problems in reading or writing may represent a great loss if his/her occupation happens to be writing.

It is also important to consider the effect of communication difficulties on a person's carers and loved ones. Communication is a two-way process, so an individual's communication problem becomes a family problem.

Carers will also feel frustration and loss in being unable to communicate with or help the person with a communication disorder. There will be changes of role and altered responsibilities for family members, and relationships may suffer as a result of these changes. Not only will there be social and emotional effects, but there may be significant financial and practical concerns.

Assessment and management of communication disorders

Communication disorders need to be assessed in depth over a period of time. **Speech and language therapists (see page 171) are the only professionals who are trained to do this and anyone presenting with a communication disorder should be referred to a speech and language therapist for assessment and advice.**

There is an increasing amount of research evidence concerning the outcomes and efficacy of speech and language therapy. For example, a list of efficacy studies for dysphasia is available from the support group Action for Dysphasic Adults (see page 28, Section 2: Factfile: Dysphasia for address).

There is rarely a 'cure' for communication disorders of neurological origin. However, much can be done to advise the patients and carers about ways in which to make best use of whatever communication is still available. Understanding more about the nature of the problems and how best to cope with them is crucial to the support of both patient and carers.

Following assessment, a speech and language therapist may recommend treatment using either individual or group therapy. For some of the progressive disorders, 'bursts' of therapy might be the most effective management. Therapy can be delivered in hospital, home, clinic or nursing home, according to local resources. The speech and language therapist will monitor a client's progress and re-assess his or her needs over time. This may include the recommendation to develop alternative means of communication as a disorder progresses.

For many people who present with communication problems, the problems will remain a long term disability and families will need as much long term support as possible. Provision will vary according to district, but speech and language therapists work very closely with other support agencies (e.g. local stroke clubs, local branches of the Stroke Association, Motor Neurone Disease Association, Parkinson's Disease Society, Alzheimer's Disease Society) to try to develop the most effective individual support systems.

Referral to and involvement of these agencies will be recommended as appropriate.

FURTHER READING

Stroke - questions and answers - S1

Learning to speak again - S2

Both published by the Stroke Association.

How to help the dysphasic person

A series of five booklets published by Action for Dysphasic Adults.

Living with Parkinson's Disease

Published by the Parkinson's Disease Society.

Motor Neurone Disease: Speech Impairment - Leaflet No 8

Published by the Motor Neurone Disease Association.

The addresses of all the charities listed above are given in Section 2: Factfile under the relevant disease or condition. Further addresses can be found in Section 6: Some Useful Addresses.

Eating and drinking

Difficulties in swallowing and the practical aspects of eating and drinking are problems which develop in some neurological disorders. These conditions can be distressing and in some cases life threatening. They need early assessment, intervention and regular review, especially in progressive disorders.

TYPES OF SWALLOWING DIFFICULTIES

Swallowing difficulties fall into two categories, those which relate specifically to neuromuscular disorders (true dysphagic disorders) and general eating and drinking problems. Both types of problems will affect nutritional levels but the management of them will be different.

- True dysphagic disorders

  These disorders usually correspond to the three (conventionally described) stages of swallowing:

  ~ **Oral difficulties**, which are the result of weakness or reduced range of oral movement. The patient may have difficulty in forming a cohesive bolus and transferring it from the front to the back of the mouth. Reduced lip movement may cause food or drink to spill from the mouth. If there is reduced tongue movement or oral pressure, there may not be sufficient movement from the front to the back of the mouth to trigger the next stages of swallowing.

  ~ **Pharyngeal difficulties**, where neurological damage causes delay in triggering the swallow reflex. The uncoordinated transfer of the bolus of food and ineffective swallowing may lead to aspiration, especially with thin fluids. Where

laryngeal elevation and movement of the soft palate are reduced and the vocal cords do not close sufficiently, the airway is not protected and there is a danger of aspiration. Weak pharyngeal movement and reduced peristalsis may add to the problem.
~ **Oesophageal difficulties.** At this stage in the swallowing process, movement is involuntary and relies upon peristalsis and gravity. If peristalsis is reduced or if there are structural difficulties in the oesophagus or stomach, swallowing difficulties may arise causing reflux or regurgitation.

Aspiration is always a possibility in true dysphagic disorders. Practitioners should be alerted to this if there is:
~ Weak or absent cough reflex
~ Weak or absent swallow reflex
~ Weak or absent gag reflex
~ Weak voice
Aspiration may be indicated by: recurrent chest infections, spiking temperatures, weight loss and skin breakdown.

- General eating and drinking problems
These problems are not neuromuscular in origin. They tend to arise as a result of a person's motivation, concentration, posture, awareness, mood and the practical aspects of eating.

Management of eating and swallowing problems

The fear of choking or starving may be of real concern to both the person with the problem and his/her family carer/s. It is essential therefore that they are both given support and advice on how best to manage their particular types of problems.

If the onset of eating and swallowing problems is

recent and sudden as in the case of stroke, regular assessment and treatment can result in significant improvements in swallowing.

In progressive disorders, regular review will help to prepare the person for new and increasing problems and help him/her to maintain higher levels of skill to cope with them.

If a patient is suspected of having difficulty in swallowing s/he should be referred to a speech and language therapist (see page 171) who will:

- Assess oral movement, safety reflexes and skills at each stage of swallowing with different consistencies of food and liquid. A videofluoroscopy (modified barium meal) may also be necessary to provide further objective measurement.
- Treat and advise the patient, the family/carers and other members of the multidisciplinary team on the best way to manage the problem.

This assessment may also include a specialist dietary or nutritional assessment or review.

Where the problems relate to the oral or pharyngeal stages of swallowing, the speech and language therapist will recommend and implement measures for managing the problems. These may include:

- Modifying the diet - for example a soft diet and thickened liquids for someone with oral and pharyngeal problems may help to prevent aspiration
- Specific exercises, for example to improve tongue and lip movements
- Changing posture - for example, turning the head to compensate for weakness on one side of the pharynx; positioning food to compensate for weakness in the mouth
- Teaching the person techniques to increase safety,

for example, double swallowing
- Supervising eating to remind the person to chew, swallow and cough if and when necessary
- Varying food temperature and taste to stimulate swallowing
- Providing advice such as: eat a little and often; take time over eating; avoid talking and eating.
- Practical issues such as: making sure the plate is conveniently positioned; personal preferences are met; false teeth fit well

Many of these measures will be carried out by the patient and family carers under the guidance of the speech and language therapist.

If nutritional levels are not being maintained, the primary care team will need to consider alternative methods of feeding. However there are ethical issues involved concerning the person's right to choose not to eat and their involvement in the process of deciding which alternative methods of feeding should be used.[1,2]

References

1. Burgess, A. (1994a) Dilemmas of deglutition. *Bulletin of the Royal College of Speech & Language Therapists,* **508,** 4 - 5.

2. Burgess, A. (1994b) Nasogastric or gastrostomy feeding? *Bulletin of the Royal College of Speech & Language Therapists,* **512,** 6 - 7.

Further reading

Logemann, J.A. (1983) *Evaluation and Treatment of Swallowing Disorders.* College Hill Press, San Diego.

Groher, M.E. (1992) *Dysphagia: Diagnosis and Management.* Butterworth Heinemann, Boston.

Swallowing difficulties after stroke. Stroke Association.
Living with Parkinson's Disease. Parkinson's Disease Society.

Parkinson's Disease Information Pack. Parkinson's Disease Society.

Motor Neurone Disease: Eating, drinking and associated difficulties. Motor Neurone Disease Association.

Addresses of these organisations can be found in Section 6: Some Useful Addresses.

Insomnia

Insomnia is a difficult symptom to define, so the first step when someone complains of not being able to sleep is to find out exactly what s/he means.

The first paragraph in the hypnotics section of the British National Formulary[1], p.149, says: '...it should be noted that some patients have unrealistic sleep expectations...'.

It is important to remember that one person's 'hardly slept a wink' is another's 'reasonable night'.

It is then important to ask the patient what s/he thinks is causing the insomnia.

The most common causes include:

- An uncomfortable bed
- Unsuitable bedclothes
- Being too hot or too cold
- Noise, lights
- Symptoms such as pain, muscle cramp, frequency of micturition
- Worry, anxiety, fear
- Disturbing dreams

Other causes might be:

- Medication which may interfere with sleep, for example caffeine, corticosteroids or diuretics, particularly if taken in the evening
- Boredom
- Sleeping during the day
- Clinical depression

Many common causes of insomnia are treatable without recourse to hypnotic or anxiolytic drugs.

A patient who is suffering from insomnia can also affect his or her carer's sleep patterns. This can increase the carer's stress levels and lead to physical and mental exhaustion if it occurs over a long period of time (see page 144: Supporting the Carers).

MANAGEMENT OF INSOMNIA

Finding out what patient and carer consider to be the consequences of the patient 'not sleeping' will provide information about the physical and emotional impact the insomnia is having on the household and the urgency of addressing it (see page 119: Dependency).

Armed with knowledge of the situation and the views of patient and carer, logical management involves:

- Addressing any environmental problems, for example: uncomfortable bed, noise
- Addressing any physical, emotional and/or psychological problems (see pages 114 and 127: Coping; Emotional States)
- Reviewing current medication and its timing before prescribing anxiolytic or hypnotic drugs

THE USE OF DRUGS

Antidepressant drugs have been widely found to be effective in the management of chronic pain, both in people with and without clinically recognisable depression. For example, amitriptyline 25 mg at night is the single most effective treatment for post herpetic neuralgia.

Skeletal muscle relaxants can relieve nocturnal muscle cramps and chronic spasticity, which are common causes of insomnia (see page 111: Pain).

Hypnotics and anxiolytics are convenient and widely prescribed in the treatment of insomnia. However, the rapid development of tolerance as well as physical and psychological dependence is a major drawback in their use. It has been recorded that dependence on these drugs develops in just a few weeks.

The British National Formulary[1],states the drugs in these categories 'should be reserved for short courses to alleviate acute conditions after causal factors have been established.' (p.150)

In practice, identification and treatment of the causes of insomnia successfully alleviate the condition in a high proportion of people.

REFERENCE

1. *British National Formulary: No 30* (1996) BMA and the Royal Pharmaceutical Company of Great Britain.

Mobility

Losing the ability to move, and hence physical independence, can have the most profound effect not only on the individual concerned, but also on the lives of his or her family, carer and friends.

Loss of mobility due to neurological damage may be sudden or gradual depending on the condition.

Movements previously taken for granted may become impossible affecting the person's functional ability, skills, appearance and body image. This can impact on their relationships with others especially their carers.

Negative images of helplessness and dependency are exacerbated by social attitudes to disability and a society organised around able-bodied people.

Early intervention by a physiotherapist is vital in order to:

- **Help a person regain or maintain mobility**
- **Prevent further problems occurring**
- **Speed possible recovery**

The physiotherapist can help people to:

- **Understand normal body movements**
- **Accept that the disease process in progressive conditions cannot be delayed**
- **Learn new skills to compensate for reduced function**
- **Maintain a positive body image**

Disorders of movement

Disorders of movement caused by disturbance of the central nervous system are associated with an increase or decrease in postural tone, abnormal co-ordination of muscle action and inadequate or faulty assimilation. The following problems can result:

- Loss of balance, including difficulties in adjusting and maintaining balance, particularly when the person is in the upright position
- Loss of stability, where the person is no longer able to stabilise one part of the body in order to enable another part to move selectively and skillfully
- Loss of perception, which may cause a person to exaggerate movements in search of a reference point, neglect affected areas of the body, or exhibit behavioural difficulties which may be interpreted as a lack of motivation or co-operation

Disorders of functional mobility

The inability to co-ordinate movement creates major problems for people in carrying out normal activities of daily living such as dressing, bathing, going to the toilet and feeding themselves.

Common problems include:

- Inco-ordination
- Difficulty in initiating movement
- Difficulty transferring weight
- Freezing - being unable to move
- Fatigue from struggling in order to try to disguise these difficulties

These can result in difficulties in the following areas:

Walking The person is unable to walk rhythmically and automatically while carrying out other activities or responding to other stimuli.

Mobility in bed Difficulty in moving in bed can affect

sexual relations and the sleep patterns of both the sufferer and his/her partner.

Transfers It may be difficult to transfer safely to and from bed, chair, toilet and cars.

People often try to disguise difficulties with movement and may struggle without help or advice longer than they should in order to 'appear normal' or 'not to give in'.

THE PHYSICAL EFFECTS OF IMMOBILITY

Weight bearing when sitting and standing is essential in maintaining normal tone, muscle length and kidney drainage.

Immobility which is not corrected can cause:

- Contractures and deformity
- Incontinence
- Pressure sores
- Oedema
- Respiratory difficulties
- Osteoporosis
- Joint pain

FACILITATING NORMAL MOVEMENT

Most neurological conditions are complex and require long term management strategies rather than ad hoc or crisis intervention.

The method most often used by physiotherapists to help people experience and relearn normal movement involves encouraging repetitive functional patterns of movement and activities. As unwanted movement decreases the person becomes more skilled in normal movement.

Other approaches used include:

- Stimulation through touch.
- Correct positioning and posture when sitting, standing and lying, with the opportunity to alter postural tone and exercise balance reactions, helps control the physical effects of immobility.
- Medication to reduce spasm, slow movement, rigidity and tremor can be effective but this in itself is not enough. People then need physiotherapy to help them make full use of their new capabilities and improve their mobility.

THE USE OF AIDS

People who are unable to move themselves may need special aids to help them achieve an acceptable level of independence.

Getting in and out of bed can be made easier with the correct use of, for example, a rope ladder. For someone who is very immobile, an adjustable bed may be an option.

Transfers can be assisted by: positioning and adjusting the height of furniture, installing a shower and the use of equipment such as sliding boards, bath boards, turntables and hoists.

The need for walking aids is assessed by a physiotherapist and provided by the NHS on a short term basis. Wheelchairs are available through the NHS, but electric wheelchairs for outdoor use have to be funded privately or through charitable sources.

Aids needed for long term use are usually available following assessment by an occupational therapist from the social services department (see Section 4: page 163). Responsibility for long term provision varies according to the area. It may lie with the social services, with the NHS, or jointly.

While mobility aids can and often do have an immediate effect in improving a person's independence, used incorrectly they can cause long term problems such as:

- Asymmetry and orientation away from the affected side if a unilateral support is used, which may lead to the development of or an increase in spasticity
- A decrease in balance reactions because head and trunk movements are reduced
- Changed posture as weight is transferred to the support
- Increased trunk and hip flexion if bilateral support is used
- The affected side or limb/s may atrophy through lack of use

It is important that a physiotherapist regularly assesses a person's needs, provides information, advises on the most appropriate types of aids, and monitors progress.

EFFECTS ON THE CARERS

Attention should not be focused solely on the person whose mobility is affected. Family carers will also need advice about handling skills and the use of equipment in order to maximise the person's ability and avoid injury.

There is a constant fear that the disabled person may fall or be harmed. This causes tension and anxiety and may in fact increase the possibility of an accident.

Regulations on handling patients were introduced in 1991 to protect hospital employees from injury. However family carers are not trained to avoid injury despite the fact that many care for people who have increasing problems with mobility in unfavourable environments.

Carers may themselves be unfit but often struggle until a crisis occurs before seeking help.

Regular assessment of both patient and carer would help to prevent problems and avoid crisis intervention.

Physiotherapists working with occupational therapists (see pages 166 - 170: Section 4) can advise carers on:

- How to help a person get up from the floor
- Coping strategies that can allay fears and reduce the risk of falls
- Particular movement problems and handling skills to help improve mobility and avoid personal injury
- Handling equipment such as philislides, turntables, and hoists to eliminate lifting
- Environmental changes such as ramps, stair lifts, commodes and positioning furniture to reduce physical effort
- Time management and the need for respite

DRIVING

Car drivers have a legal responsibility to inform the DVLA and their insurers of any disability, if it is going to last more than 3 months and affects their ability to drive or could do so in the future.

- Assessment
  - ~ A range of assessments of wheelchair users and car drivers are carried out at ten accredited mobility centres located throughout the country (see page 211).
  - ~ All accredited centres have adapted cars to test drive and some have powered wheelchairs and scooters.

~ There is an assessment fee but assessment minimises the risk of buying an unsuitable vehicle.

~ Every other year the Department of Transport Information Service (MAVIS, see page 211-12) organises a mobility road show at Crowthorne in Berkshire where different cars with various adaptations may be test driven on private tracks.

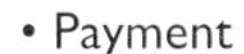

• Payment

~ People receiving the higher rate mobility component of the Disability Living Allowance may lease a car from Motability. Motability also has a hire purchase scheme for new and second hand cars and may provide assistance with the payment of specialist vehicle adaptations and driving lessons. (see page 211: Section 6: Some Useful Addresses).

~ Value Added Tax (VAT) may be zero rated for appliances and accessories designed for or used by disabled people. This may include new vehicles but only if they are modified for a person to drive or travel whilst seated in a wheelchair and the modifications are carried out before the vehicle is registered. (Further information regarding VAT may be obtained from local HM Customs and Excise offices.)

~ People receiving the higher rate mobility component of the Disability Living Allowance who have a vehicle mainly for their own use may be exempt from road tax. Information can be obtained from the DVLA and the Department of Transport leaflet V188.

• Insurance

~ People with disabilities are often expected to pay more for motor insurance so are advised to shop around for the best deal or seek advice from their local Motability centre.

Fitness to drive is assessed by the patient's GP, according to the guidelines laid down by the Driver and Vehicle Licensing Authority in the booklet: *At a Glance Guide to the Current Medical Standards of Fitness to Drive* (DVLA, Swansea: March 1996).

Further reading

Bobath, B. (1970) *Adult Hemiplegia; Evaluation and Treatment.* Heinemann, London.

Carr, J., Shepherd, R. (1990) *Physiotherapy in Disorders of the Brain.* Butterworth Heinemann, Oxford.

Cotton, E., Kinsman, R. (1989) *Conductive Education for Adult Hemiplegia.* Churchill Livingstone, Edinburgh.

Darnborough, A., Kirkdale, D. (1991) *Motoring and Mobility for Disabled people.* RADAR. (Now out of print - new edition March 1997.)

Davies, P. (1985) *Steps to Follow. A Guide to the Treatment of Adult Hemiplegia.* Springer-Verlag, Berlin

Dept. of Transport *Door to Door. Transport for People with Disabilities.* HMSO, London. (Updated every 2-3 years - advice about benefits and allowances - planning journeys local and far afield, including travel abroad - lots of useful addresses e.g. Stroke Association.)

Kidd, J., Lawes, N., Musa, I. (1992) *Understanding Neuromuscular Plasticity, a basis for clinical rehabilitation.* Edward Arnold - division of Hodder and Stoughton, London.

Mandlestam, M. (1993) *How to Get Equipment for Disability.* Disabled Living Foundation. Jessica Kingsley Publishers and Kogan Page, London. 3rd edn.

Swain, J., Finklestein, V., French, S., Oliver, M. (1993) *Disabling Barriers Enabling Environment.* OU Press/Sage publications, London.

Chronic pain

Pain is a common symptom, and its control has been a primary objective of 'healers' throughout the centuries.

Where pain is a presenting symptom, the usual procedure is to identify the site, severity and history of the pain in order to diagnose the cause before starting treatment.

However in people with persistent neurological conditions, pain tends to be chronic and can be easily overlooked. Investigation and assessment of this chronic pain are rarely made.

In people with chronic neurological conditions, it is easy to overlook the fact that they may suffer with chronic pain.

The pain associated with neurological conditions usually has a physical, pathological basis. However, the severity of the pain the person experiences is greatly influenced by other physical, emotional or psycho-social factors.

An uncomfortable bed or chair, an overheated or cold environment can lower the pain threshold. Anxiety, fear, anger, depression and boredom can have the same effect. Lack of sleep and tiredness also reduce the pain threshold leading to low morale and misery.

Few analgesic drugs will be fully effective in the presence of these additional contributory factors.

Before attempting pain relief with drugs, it is essential to consider the extent to which factors which lower the pain threshold exist.

People with neurological conditions rarely volunteer the fact that they are living with chronic pain: 'It's all part of it' and 'If it was important the doctor would ask...' are comments commonly reported by nurses caring for such patients.

Family carers of people with chronic pain may be equally reluctant to volunteer their own worries, depression and exhaustion. The onus for raising the subject therefore often lies with the doctor or nurse.

Continuing pain needs continuing treatment and review of both patient and carer.

Management of pain

The commonest causes of chronic pain in people with neurological conditions arise as a side effect of the condition rather than from a disorder of nervous tissue itself. For example:

- Shoulder pain may result from subluxation of the joint in the arm paralysed by a stroke
- Patients may suffer painful contractures if they do not receive physiotherapy and active nursing care
- Muscular cramps are common in the early stages of Parkinson's disease

Management of such conditions involves: recognising the pain exists; identifying the cause; providing 24-hour pain relief; regular review and assessment.

Treatment will depend on the cause and ideally should begin early enough to prevent chronic pain developing (prevention of the contractures following stroke is a good example).

Once chronic pain is present the logical sequence is to:

- Confirm the cause

- Identify any factors which may raise or lower the pain threshold
- Collaborate with colleagues to try and eliminate/minimise these factors
- Consider the possibility of therapy within primary care. This might involve one or more of the following:
  - ~ Medication directed at the cause of the pain and relevant to the type and severity of the pain. The conventional approach to relieving pain whose cause is not reversible is to move up the ladder starting with aspirin, paracetamol and dihydrocodeine; move on through non-steroidal anti-inflammatory drugs and phenazocine; and finally use morphia and other agonist opioids.
  - ~ Skeletal muscle relaxants, including dantrolene, baclofen, diazepam and quinine salts may be useful in relieving cramps provided care is taken over possible side effects such as an increase in muscle tone impairment and therefore an increase in the degree of disability.
  - ~ Alternative pain relief such as TENS (Transcutaneous Electrical Nerve Stimulation), acupuncture or hypnotherapy.
  - ~ Physiotherapy.
- Decide whether specialist help is needed from, for example: a pain clinic, rehabilitation unit or palliative care team

It may be helpful if the pain pathways are interrupted chemically, using for example, intrathecal therapy, or physically, using for example, cryoanalgesia.

When assessing people with chronic neurological conditions, chronic pain needs to be identified and treated seriously.

Coping

'Coping' refers to the various ways (thoughts as well as behaviours) in which people actually respond to a stressful situation, so as to resolve the problem and/or relieve the associated distress.

People experiencing neurological conditions, and their carers, can have a great deal to cope with:

- Physical difficulties and limitations
- Disturbing behaviours
- Loss of work and sense of identity
- Isolation and alienation
- Communication difficulties
- Financial problems
- Forming and sustaining meaningful relationships
- Difficult emotional states (see page 127: Emotional States)
- The need for both sufferers and carers to be flexible to meet different needs and demands as the condition changes or deteriorates over time

How do people cope?

There are adaptive ways of coping that can be recommended and supported by health care professionals, and more maladaptive ways of coping that they should be on the alert for and assist those involved to avoid if possible.

- Coping is a conscious process that can be described, reflected upon and modified by the person involved, and which can be observed or elicited through questioning by an observer.
- Coping can consist of a complex number of responses aimed at meeting the different stresses

that may be associated with the conditions. Coping with a stroke, for example, may mean coping with such specific aspects as paralysis, feelings of frustration and depression, altered perception, disturbed communication, loss of work and role within the family, changed relationships, and balancing needs for independence with increased dependency.

- Some people will cope with certain aspects better than others. Carers often find disturbed behaviour (for example, irritability, constant demands, resistiveness, night-time disturbance) in their loved one more difficult to cope with than physical dependency needs such as help with dressing or washing.

One common way of describing coping is in terms of 'problem-focused' and 'emotion-focused' coping.

- Problem-focused coping refers to ways of coping that aim to identify the particular problem(s) causing distress, generate appropriate solutions that will resolve the problem(s), and implement these.
- Emotion-focused coping involves first accepting that a given problem cannot be completely or perhaps even partially resolved. The aim is then to modify or change the associated distress by, for example: using relaxation or other stress management techniques; refocusing on activities or events which may evoke positive feelings such as pleasure, satisfaction or mastery so that the distress is minimised or kept in perspective.
- These two ways of coping can themselves be broken down into a number of different strategies, such as information seeking, social support seeking,

focusing on positive events and experiences, cognitive reframing.

They are not mutually exclusive, and may be used together in coping with any given stressful situation; for example, managing stress or frustration through relaxation techniques while working out a way to resolve a problem.

However, sometimes one approach is more appropriate than another and care has to be taken that the correct balance is achieved. Health care professionals can have an important role in monitoring the use of coping strategies by patients and carers alike, and in taking steps to ensure that people are not 'stuck' in using one approach inappropriately (for example, continually trying to 'problem-solve' an unresolvable problem when they would be better advised to focus on coping with the associated distress).

Avoidance coping

There are more maladaptive ways of coping and these often involve some long term use of avoidance coping strategies, such as ignoring problems in the hope that they will go away, wishful thinking, or taking the line of least resistance in the hope that things will sort themselves out.

- Sometimes the 'head in the sand' approach is appropriate, especially if the stress is acute and will pass. If, however, the stress is chronic and recurring, avoidance coping alone is often associated with increased stress.
- The use of formal carers' support services may inadvertently reinforce avoidance coping. For example, when respite care is used as the only way of helping a carer cope with a loved one's disturbing behaviour it may help to defuse an acute crisis but

may only buy limited time and relief. In such cases, respite care needs to be considered in the context of helping the carer and loved one cope more directly with the difficult behaviour and associated distress.

If used as the principal means of coping with chronic and unremitting difficulties, avoidance coping can be associated with increased stress levels. It may 'buy time' in the short term, but does not resolve the problem.

DEVELOPING COPING SKILLS: THE ROLE OF THE HEALTH CARE PROFESSIONAL

The development of appropriate coping skills can reduce levels of stress in both the person with the condition and the carer. This can be achieved through:

- One-to one work with individuals
- Working with couples and families
- Group work where people with similar problems, carers and sufferers, may meet on a regular basis - perhaps eventually becoming a self-help group

The development of coping skills is often collaborative and may involve:

- Information provision: this in itself can be a real skill in terms of judging the right sort of information for any given individual(s); presenting it at the right time, and in the right way.
- Helping people to develop and practise problem-solving skills, learn appropriate stress management techniques, and increase awareness of unhelpful coping strategies - in particular those that may be based on avoidance strategies alone.
- Developing an appropriate level of social support.

More information about the roles that different professionals can play in helping people cope with neurological disease and disability can be found in Section 4: Psychological Support (page 157), and also the relevant Factsheets in Section 2: Factfile. It should be remembered, however, that coping does not stand alone and should always be seen within the context of good overall service provision.

Dependency

National figures show that of the 6.5 million people in the UK with disability about half have relatively minor non-progressive problems while the other half are severely or very severely disabled, and as a consequence are unable to live independently.

Most people with incurable neurological disease become increasingly dependent before they die.

The process of becoming dependent may be slow, for example, for most people who have Parkinson's disease; more rapid, for example, in the case of motor neurone disease; or instantaneous, for example, with most people who have a stroke.

The onset and development of dependency can result in a major life change both for the dependent person and for the domestic carer, family, friend or neighbour who is involved in providing support (see also page 114: Coping, and page 127: Emotional States).

In managing primary care, it is essential to be aware of the aspects of life in which a disabled person is dependent, and to know who is providing the disabled person with support at home.

TYPES OF DEPENDENCY

Aspects of life in which people with neurological disease may become dependent vary according to:

- The disease and its severity
- The ways in which the disease affects each individual
- Each individual's character and personality
- The character and personality of the family carers

Dependence can occur in one area but is more usually in multiple and related areas. It often begins, before the development of chronic symptoms, with a psychological dependence on others based on fear and loss of confidence in a person with a newly-diagnosed condition. As symptoms develop, this moves into:

- Physical dependence, which is common and easily recognised. It is usually caused by loss of function of voluntary muscles, and it may result in inability to carry out any activities of normal daily life due to loss of mobility (see also page 103: Mobility, page 89: Communication and page 95: Swallowing).
- Physical disability and dependence can in turn give rise to emotional and psychological dependence with the disabled person relying on carers for constant understanding and emotional support.
- Mental dependence occurs when the disabled person loses the ability to remember, orientate and reason. Mental deterioration can lead to restlessness, wandering and behavioural changes including aggression.
- Social dependence is very common in people with advanced disabling neurological disease of whatever cause. Loss of function means that they become dependent, often totally, on domestic carers to organise transport, to interpret what they are trying to say and to ensure they are socially acceptable.

Consequences of dependency

The onset and steady advance of dependency can have severe physical, emotional, psychological, mental and social effects on both the person and the carer.

As the disease progresses and the disabled person becomes less able to do things for him/herself it is usual for the family carer to become 'locked-in' to the situation.

At the same time, the guilt, anger, frustration and often fear which increase in the disabled person are often mirrored by similar emotions in the family carer. Fear of the future and of not being able to cope are common. Changing roles and relationships are often difficult to handle (see page 131: Psycho-sexual Problems). Anxiety and depression frequently occur.

When in addition the family carer is responsible for 'turning' the disabled person in bed or helping him or her on to a commode day and night, often involving heavy physical exertion; is involved in dressing and feeding; is obliged to carry out many intimate tasks; and is him/herself affected by loss of sleep, loss of social contacts and by isolation, it is not surprising that when asked how they feel, carers may describe themselves as exhausted or as 'living in a prison'.

Identification of the needs and provision of support for the family carers who play a key role in caring for dependent people at home is an essential component of management (see page 144: Supporting the Carers).

Measuring dependency

In managing the care of a dependent person at home, it is a great advantage to be able to measure the degree of dependency and the amount of strain experienced by the domestic carer. By using the same measures for review on a regular basis, changes in the situation can be recognised and appropriate management decisions made to cater for these changes.

Although a number of physical disability scales, mental test scores and activities of daily living assessment scales have been devised, no single scale relating to dependence is as yet generally accepted.

However, in a number of projects undertaken in general practice, three scales of dependency have been found to be relevant and easy to administer.

1 The Barthel Index (Figure 1) is an activity of daily living (ADL) scale, which measures the extent to which the person being assessed needs help in performing 10 common activities.
2 The Hodkinson Abbreviated Mental Test Score (Figure 2) Care must be taken when using this test to allow the person being tested sufficient time to think through the question before answering. The person undergoing the test needs to have good verbal skills for the test to be reliable. People with communication disorders could score low whatever their level of dependency. A reliable score of six or less signifies dementia.
3 The Betsy Robinson Caregiver Strain Index (Figure 3) This is a simple validated scale based on 13 items or situations which if present are likely to cause strain to domestic carers. A score of seven or more suggests high levels of strain on the carer.

It is vital to the effective management of care that professionals should develop a continuous and co-ordinated approach to monitoring domestic situations involving a patient and a family carer. The onset or development of dependency can then be recognised, and appropriate decisions made involving the whole team, the disabled person and the family carer.

Figure 1 The Barthel ADL Index

Function	Score
Feeding	
Unable	0
Needs help cutting, spreading, etc	1
Independent (food within reach)	2
Transferring	
Unable - no sitting balance	0
Major help (1-2 people), can sit	1
Minor help (physical, verbal)	2
Independent	3
Grooming	
Needs help with personal care	0
Independent (face, hair, teeth, shave)	1
Mobility	
Immobile	0
Wheelchair dependent	1
Walks with help - one person	2
Independent (± aid e.g. stick)	3
Dressing	
Dependent	0
Needs help - about 1/2 unaided	1
Independent (including buttons, zips)	2
Stairs	
Unable	0
Needs help (verbal, physical)	1
Independent (up and down)	2
Bathing	
Dependent	0
Independent (or in shower)	1

→

Function	**Score**
Bowels	
Incontinent (or enema)	0
Occasional accident (once a week)	1
Continent	2
Bladder	
Incontinent (or catheter, can't manage)	0
Occasional accident (max. once 24 hrs)	1
Continent > 7 days	2
Toilet	
Dependent	0
Needs some help	1
Independent (wiping, dressing)	2
Total Score	———

A score of 20 indicates independence; 15-19 mild loss of function; 10 - 14 moderate loss of function, 5-9 severe loss of function; 0-4 very severe loss of function.

From Collin, C., Wade, D.T., Davies, S., Horne, V. (1988) *The Barthel ADL Index:* a reliability study. *International Disability Studies,* **10,** 61-63.

Figure 2
The Hodkinson Abbreviated Mental Test Score

		Tick if correct
1	Age of subject	☐
2	Time (nearest hour)	☐
3	An address *(NB to be repeated by subject at end of test)*	☐
4	Year	☐
5	This address (i.e. name of place where subject is)	☐
6	Recognition of two persons	☐
7	Date of birth	☐
8	Year First World War started	☐
9	Name of present king/queen	☐
10	Count backwards 20 - 1	☐
3	*Recall address*	☐

Total score ——

From Hodkinson, H.M. (1972) Evaluation of a mental test score for assessment of mental impairment in the elderly. *Age and Ageing,* **1,** 233-238.

COMMON PROBLEMS 3

Figure 3 Caregiver Strain Index

	YES	NO
Sleep is disturbed	☐	☐
Have to do such a lot for him/her - takes up a lot of time	☐	☐
It is a physical strain for me	☐	☐
It stops me going out	☐	☐
Our usual life has been disrupted	☐	☐
We can't do things we used to (e.g. holiday, take a job)	☐	☐
There have been other demands on my time - conflicts with other interests	☐	☐
There have been emotional problems (e.g. arguments)	☐	☐
Some of his/her behaviour is upsetting	☐	☐
He/she has changed so much from him/her former self - upsetting	☐	☐
There have had to be adjustments in work and social life - have had to give things up	☐	☐
It is a financial strain	☐	☐
Feeling completely overwhelmed e.g. worry	☐	☐

Total Score ______

Each 'Yes' response = one

From Robinson, B. (1983) Validation of a Care-giver Strain Index. *Journal of Gerontology,* **18:3,** 344-348.

Emotional states

An individual's emotional reaction to a long term neurological condition depends on many factors, including:

- Age
- Whether the condition is present from birth or acquired
- Whether the condition is stable or progressive
- The type of symptoms presenting such as pain, disfigurement, communication difficulties, cognitive impairment, physical limitations
- The social support system which is available

As a person born with a neurological condition grows older, he or she is faced with many problems and challenges. In the context of a society which holds many negative attitudes and misconceptions concerning 'handicap', particular difficulties can recur in defining oneself and forming relationships

For a person with an acquired neurological condition, such as a stroke, there can be sudden, and sometimes emotionally overwhelming transition from 'normality' to being disabled. The task of redefining oneself and one's relationships to others, adjusting and adapting to the enormous changes that have been brought to one's life can be formidable.

Where the neurological condition is progressive, as in Parkinson's disease or motor neurone disease, there can be a continual need to reassess and readapt to changing circumstances.

Many of those who live with neurological conditions, and their carers, experience clinically significant levels of distress.

Common emotional reactions

Emotional reactions to a chronic neurological condition or disease can include:

- A sense of grief as the person comes to terms with the change from the person s/he once was, or the kind of person s/he can never be
- Depression in relation to the many losses that may be incurred in, for example: work, social role, relationships, faculties, skills and abilities, independence, hobbies and interests
- Anxiety in relation to uncertainty about new challenges as well as learning how to face and cope with many of the activities and routine tasks of daily life that are ordinarily taken for granted
- Helplessness at being unable to resolve problems
- Frustration, bitterness and despair as s/he tries to come to terms with the sense of unfairness at what has happened

Effects on carers

Carers can also experience these emotions as well as feelings of burden, guilt and self-blame. For example, it has been estimated that 25-33 per cent of all stroke survivors may be clinically depressed at any one time, and one study found that as many as 67 per cent of stroke carers may have significant levels of distress.

The lack of recognition or under-treatment of heightened emotional states can be a common cause of failure or poor progress in rehabilitation.

Assessing emotional problems

Assessment of emotional status is an important part of the total assessment, and should be done on a continuous and co-ordinated basis by whichever members of the multidisciplinary care team are most involved with the patient and the carer (see Section 4). Emotional states can strongly influence both physical and psychological symptoms (see page 111: Pain, and page 100: Insomnia).

People need time and opportunity to talk about their feelings as well as their physical problems and symptoms.

- Sometimes people living with these conditions and their family carers find it difficult to express their feelings directly, finding it easier to present with and talk about multiple or vague physical symptoms which may conceal other problems.
- At other times, emotional reactions may be distorted by the defences and coping mechanisms people employ when stressed (see page 114: Coping). In these circumstances distress may show itself as anger and hostility, non-compliance, withdrawal (often mistaken for 'poor motivation'), denial, projection and blaming others, and excessive dependency. Understanding the emotional problems underlying these behaviours may be challenging for the practitioner.
- Clarifying the presence and severity of anxiety or depression may be carried out through interview and/or perhaps the use of one of the many self-report screening questionnaires that are available (for example, the Hospital Anxiety and Depression Scale[1]).
- For those unable to communicate, there may be behavioural indicators such as emotional lability, withdrawal, lack of eye contact, agitation and restlessness, poor concentration or bodily tension, or someone close to the person can answer questions about whether they feel the individual is distressed.

Appropriate help and support for those sufferers and carers experiencing debilitating distress depends very much on the individual, the severity of distress, and whether the problem is long or short term.

- The knowledge that there is an interested and caring professional to turn to is a powerful preventive and ameliorative measure.
- Provision of appropriate and sensitive information aids understanding and hence self-coping is very important.
- Giving practical advice will help people access the services they need.
- Peer support, as in local branches of national support groups (see the addresses in the relevant Factsheets in Section 2), enables people with the condition and their family and carers to draw advice and ideas from others who have similar experiences to theirs. However, not everyone is a 'group' person, so this type of support may not always be appropriate.

- Formal therapy, as provided by clinical psychologists, for example, may help some find ways of managing stress and depressed mood and to adjust/adapt to their condition. Some may benefit from less formal counselling (see page 157: Psychological support). Others may need to consider the short term use of psychotropic medications initially and perhaps in addition to other approaches.

REFERENCE

1. Zimond, A.S., Snaith, R.P. (1983) The Hospital Anxiety and Depression Scale. *Acta Psychiatrica Scandinavia,* **67,** 361 - 370.

Psycho-sexual problems

The concept of human sexuality embraces all those factors which result in our capacity to love and procreate. This includes the individual's perception and expression of 'womanliness' or 'manliness'.

Emotional and sexual relationships are highly significant in the lives of most people. This need for human relationships does not disappear with the onset of physical disability. It is therefore important that an individual suffering from a disabling condition acknowledges him/herself and is acknowledged by society as a sexual being with similar needs and desires to able-bodied peers.This can often be a difficult area for health care professionals, due to embarrassment and lack of understanding of the problems, combined with the reluctance of the patient and carer to discuss the subject.

Psycho-sexual problems can occur both as a direct (primary) and indirect (secondary) result of physical disability.

A survey carried out by Stewart[1] showed that 75% of people with physical disability experienced sexual and/or emotional problems, often lasting a considerable time. Of these:

- 45% were caused by physical factors
- 15% were due to psychological factors
- 36% were due to a combination of both

The greater the degree of disability, the greater the problem.

Direct effects

The direct effect of disability on sexual function means that the usual sexual response does not take place even when the individual is sexually aroused.

In men, this can result in:

- Difficulty in getting an erection
- Inability to reach orgasmic climax
- Premature ejaculation, or 'coming' too soon
- Reaching orgasm, but with reduced intensity of feeling

In women, the problems may be:

- Difficulty in having an orgasm
- Having an orgasm, but experiencing little feeling
- Vaginal dryness, making intercourse painful
- Irregular periods, or periods stopping altogether, causing anxiety and uncertainty

In both sexes:

- Physical impairment, making intercourse difficult
- Loss of feeling, or unpleasant sensitivity and pain
- Loss of the use of the hands, making foreplay and masturbation difficult
- Speech problems, making it difficult to talk about sexual needs
- Incontinence, which causes embarrassment, fear or distaste
- Tiredness and reduced physical and mental stamina, which can reduce the desire for sexual activity

Indirect effects

Where the disability exists from an early age, a person's sexual development and maturity will be affected, with limited social and sexual experience and access to sex education. This may lead to sexually inappropriate behaviour, both in the home and in public.

The secondary effects of disability on sexual functioning relate to the psychosocial response of the patient and partner to the impairment.

In the disabled person:

- Loss of feelings of physical attractiveness can result in lowered self esteem, depression, sadness and despondency.
- Recognition that someone (often the partner) is providing intimate personal care can create feelings of infantilisation, with attendant desexualisation.
- Experiencing anxiety, rejection, impatience, embarrassment, anger, avoidance from others will affect his/her self esteem and feelings of femininity or masculinity.

In the partner:

- Loss of attraction to the disabled person, because of changes in appearance, sexual behaviour, or personal grooming which the partner finds unacceptable
- Communication difficulties, particularly if the disabled person makes new demands on the partner which the partner considers inappropriate
- Anxiety and tiredness and possibly avoidance, revulsion and embarrassment, as the familiar roles of loving and caring are redefined
- Changed relationships in the family as a whole can also affect the roles of the disabled person and partner

TREATMENT

The extent to which help for sexual problems can be addressed will depend upon the nature and severity of the problem. If it is not resolved within 6-12 months, then a full recovery is unlikely.

A disabled person may experience a variety of sexual problems and for this reason it may be difficult to identify a single health care professional to approach for help. The section on psychological support services (page 157) describes some possible variations in local services and it is important for GPs to be aware of what is available to them in the local area.

Practical intervention usually takes the form of education or counselling.

- Education - appropriate to the age and experience of the patient, i.e. whether s/he is adjusting to a new set of problems (for example, following a stroke) or finding ways of living with old problems (for example, a child with a neurological disorder reaching adolescence). Measures might include:
  - ~ Practical advice about intercourse, masturbation, incontinence, alternative methods of sexual expression and the use of devices to assist sex
  - ~ Social skills training
- Counselling of the disabled person should involve discussion about fears and fantasies, feelings of infantilisation, assessing memory loss, exploring what is appropriate sexual behaviour, responsibility, birth control, sexual expression.

There are a number of ethical issues related to the treatment of psycho-sexual problems in disabled people. At the heart of these is the issue of how much control it is 'right' to exert over other people. For example, do young disabled people have the right to experience what is morally wrong?

Counselling may also be appropriate for the carer and/or partner in order to relieve stress, anxiety or guilt about their feelings, or to enable them to cope with challenging or aggressive behaviour from the disabled person. Marital therapy in the form of counselling from specialist organisations may also be available.

There are three types of organisations offering help and support on psycho-sexual problems:

• Those welcoming everyone needing guidance
• Those specialising in helping all disabled people with their relationships
• Those dedicated to particular disabilities

Details of addresses of these organisations are given in Section 6: Some Useful Addresses, under the heading Sex and personal relationships (page 206).

Reference

1. Stewart, W.F.R. (1975) *Sex and the physically handicapped.* The National Fund for Research into Crippling Disease, London.

Further reading

Goodwill C.J., Chamberlain A.M. (eds) (1988) *Rehabilitation of the physically disabled adult.* Croom Helm, London.

Social difficulties

The Department of Health has produced an extremely useful book which gives up-to-date information about the areas discussed in this section. It is called *A Practical Guide for Disabled People: where to find information, services and equipment* and is available free of charge from Department of Health, PO Box 410, Wetherby LS23 7LN. It is also available from this address as an audio cassette, and in braille.

PRACTICAL NEEDS

Where there is a need for assistance in the home, either to provide practical help, such as housework, shopping, pension collection and mobile meals, or personal care, such as help with dressing, washing, going to the toilet, and getting in and out of bed, the GP should approach social services and ask them to carry out an assessment of need. On the basis of this assessment, the social services department may offer the person some or all of the services required.

If a carer is providing a substantial amount of the care needed, he or she is also entitled to a separate assessment by social services of his or her own needs (see page 144: Supporting the Carers).

These written assessments will usually be carried out by a member of the social work staff. At the same time, they will also be able to make an assessment of whether the person or his/her carer would benefit from respite care of some sort. This could either be on a daily basis, when, for example, the person with the condition attends a day centre, or on a longer term basis, with the person receiving residential care away from the home, or with someone coming into the home to enable the carer to have a break.

If the person needs simple items of equipment, such as a raised lavatory seat, bathing equipment, rails in the bathroom or on the stairs, or major adaptations to the home to enable him or her to remain safely at home, then a social services occupational therapist will be asked to carry out an assessment as well (see page 168: Section 4).

Who should refer?

Anyone can refer a person to the social services department. A good starting point is the duty officer. The department will want confirmation that the person needing support knows s/he has been referred.

Who is eligible?

Eligibility criteria and charges for social services support are locally determined. In some areas the district nursing service will provide personal assistance, such as bathing, and smaller pieces of equipment if they are already involved in providing care.

Social needs

There are enormous, and often insurmountable, barriers to a disabled person participating in the life of the community. Many disabled people (and their carers) are socially very isolated, and this can add to both their practical and emotional problems.

A number of factors exacerbate the potential difficulties of leading a 'normal' social life experienced by those who have mobility problems, for example:

- Poverty: Large numbers of disabled people are dependent on state benefits; some are unable to work because of their impairment, others could work but do not, because of the current economic climate and/or the attitudes of employers. As part of the care management package, someone should check the person's benefit entitlement (see below).

- Lack of accessible public transport: Travelling on public transport is often impossible because of lack of level access; where there are adapted facilities, such as on long distance trains, wheelchair users have to make their bookings well in advance. Some areas have Dial a Ride schemes, or other ways of providing adapted transport, and this needs to be checked out for your area.
- Inaccessibility and lack of suitable facilities in buildings: Disabled people can be refused access to theatres or cinemas because they are seen to be a 'fire hazard'. A range of older buildings such as post offices, banks, polling stations, shops, centres for evening classes and places of entertainment are often inaccessible and the person is unable to do the ordinary, everyday things independently, or even at all, that able-bodied people take for granted.
- Negative attitudes of able-bodied people: Social activities are often restricted to those taking place in 'special' facilities such as day centres run by the local social services department or voluntary organisations. Some disabled people do not wish to relate exclusively to disabled people and feel that their individual wishes cannot be met.

FINANCIAL NEEDS: WORK

Disabled people can get help to find employment or stay in work from a variety of organisations, including Jobcentres, careers services and voluntary organisations. Education and training can also play a part (see page 204 in Section 6: Some Useful Addresses).

- The national network of Jobcentres is run by The Employment Service, which aims to offer disabled people help and advice in finding and retaining work or appropriate training, and to help and encourage employers to make work or training opportunities available to them.
- Some disabled people will also be eligible for a disability employment adviser (DEA), who works with employers and disabled people to overcome difficulties, particularly where a formerly healthy person becomes disabled and needs help in maintaining former employment. The DEA can also provide access to a range of specialised services such as help with communication, equipment for work, and so on, and advice on working from home, and supported employment schemes. Further details are given in the DoH book *A Practical Guide for Disabled People* (see page 136).

FINANCIAL NEEDS: BENEFITS

The Government acknowledges that many people do not claim the wide range of different benefits to which disabled people and their carers may be entitled. As part of the care management package, someone who knows about benefits should check that the disabled person and his or her carer are getting all they are entitled to. This can be done through the Welfare Benefits Helpline (Tel: 0800 88 22 00 or 0800 24 33 55(minicom) for people who are deaf and have a textphone) or the Local Citizen's Advice Bureau or the Welfare Benefits Advice Section of the local authority.

Benefits to which disabled people and their carers may be entitled include:

- Income Support
- Family Credit

- Disability Working Allowance
- Invalid Care Allowance
- Attendance Allowance
- Disability Living Allowance
- Severe Disablement Allowance
- Incapacity Benefit
- Housing Benefit

This list is not exhaustive, and legislation in this area is constantly changing, so you need to keep up to date.

Language and cultural needs

Access to information is a problem for everyone, but people from certain cultural groups in the community often live in greater isolation than others, especially where they speak little English.

- Those providing services should be cautious in the assumptions which they make about the needs of different cultural groups within the community. For example, it is commonly assumed by service providers that there is an extended family, particularly for Asian and Chinese families, which will invariably prefer to take the responsibility for long term care and is in a position to do this. This may be true for some, but it is far from the case for many people. The immigration process itself affects the composition of the extended family, and many aspects of life in modern Britain weaken family networks or their capacity to provide sufficient support and care.
- Similarly, it should not be assumed that because people do not come forward for services such as day care or home help that these are neither needed nor wanted. The content of services and

the ways in which they are provided may not reflect the diversity of people's needs and the realities of their lives. For example, not informing people about available respite services in their mother tongue excludes many for whom English is not their first language.

Providing a service that is responsive to the diverse needs of different sections of the community is likely to require developments in a number of different areas.

- Sensitivity and responsiveness: Service providers need to give attention to each family's circumstances when planning the services to be provided. For some families it will be critical to ensure that staff are themselves from the same cultural group as the patients and carers. Greater consultation may be needed as well as continual monitoring and review to ensure that services remain appropriate.
- Specific services: The response to supporting people from particular cultural groups is often to provide 'special' services which are seen as appropriate and helpful. However, designating these services as 'special' may contribute to the perception that people from certain cultural groups are 'problematic', requiring additional resources from an already over-stretched budget. It may be preferable to view such support as 'specific' rather than 'special'. For instance, offering a sitting service where staff members speak Punjabi, or providing a prayer room for Muslim clients in a day centre is by no means special, but is certainly a specific response.
- Providing translation: Accurately translated information on how to get services and how to complain should be given particular attention.

Complex legal jargon about benefits and procedures, or difficult medical terminology, often does not translate well. Translations should be developed in consultation with subject specialists from particular cultural groups to check that meanings are correctly conveyed

- Disseminating information: The existence of such information needs to be well publicised. Newsletters can be useful in targeting non-English-speaking people. For example, Contact a Family in Southall, Middlesex, produces a newsletter for parents in four Asian languages, providing carers with a great deal of valuable information.
- Alternatives to the written word also need to be explored. The use of ethnic community radio in some cities can offer direct contact with housebound carers whose understanding of English is limited. Audio cassette tapes, which can be played in carers' own homes, are another way of producing information. These, too, should be well publicised.
- Video films targeted at specific groups can explain a range of services to carers, for example chiropody or continence services. Some social services departments are making progress in this area and there are several informative videos aimed at the needs of specific cultural groups. For example, Leicester Council for Voluntary Services and Scope, a project for Asian elders in Leicester, have jointly developed a video for carers. Videos should be well publicised and made available for viewing in community centres, day centres and residential homes.
- Home visits may be the best way of bringing information to some carers. These could be done by people who are working with carers or by someone who speaks their language and is likely to have some understanding of their circumstances and needs.
- Use of schools: Another route for some families is

through written materials given to children to bring home from school. This may give the materials added importance and, even when in English, can be read either by someone else in the family or by a neighbour or friend.

Further reading

Atkin, K., Parker, G.M. (1993) *Community Care in a Multi-Racial Britain: A Critical Review of the Literature.* HMSO, London.

Eribo, L. (1991) *Support You Need.* Kings Fund Centre, London.

Jayaratnam, R. (1990) *Black and Ethnic Minorities Cultural Awareness.* Newham Health Authority.

Supporting the carers

Carers are people who look after relatives, friends or neighbours who could not manage to live at home without help.

- **There are almost 7 million carers in the United Kingdom**[1]
- **One in seven adults is a carer**
- **There are over 10,000 young people aged 18 and under who are carers, usually looking after a parent**
- **Many carers are older people who are themselves disabled**
- **The majority of carers are women**

THE EFFECTS OF CARING

Carers are affected by every aspect of disability, be it physical or emotional, and their need for support in dealing with the problems of disability can be as great as that of the disabled person.

It is clear from the discussion of the problems associated with disability throughout this compendium that carers' lives can be restricted in many ways by the need to take responsibility for the person for whom they are caring.

Caring for a heavily dependent person at home is often distressing, hard work and can create tensions and disruption within the family. Carers who look after someone who lives alone may have the added burden of running two homes, travelling between the two and worrying about what is happening in their absence.

Many carers find their health suffers as a result of physical and mental exhaustion and stress:

'That totally shattering feeling of tiredness - I've not had an unbroken night's sleep for 10 years.'

'After two heart attacks and a nervous breakdown, I wanted to kill my wife.' [2]

Financial hardship, social isolation and loneliness are common problems.

Supporting carers

Many people are unaware that they are carers. They may also be unaware that help and support are available and how to access it.

Carers need:

- To recognise that they are carers
- Their contribution to be recognised and valued, particularly by the primary care team
- To acknowledge their own physical, emotional, social and psychological needs, including respite
- Information and advice
- Support and access to appropriate services including appropriate respite (see page 114: Coping)

If the person for whom they are caring dies, they will continue to need support and advice as they cope with the bereavement and adjust to the change this brings to their lives. For those who have cared for a long time, this may be a difficult and painful process.

What help is available?

- Social services: from 1 April 1996, carers have a right to a separate assessment of their own ability to provide care under the Carers (Recognition and Services) Act, which states:

'The Act is concerned with carers who are either providing or intending to provide a substantial amount of care on a

regular basis. Under the Act, a carer is entitled on request to an assessment when a local authority carries out an assessment of the person cared for in respect of community care services (under Section 47 (1)(a) of NHSCCA 1990). The results of the carer's assessment should be taken into account when the local authority is making decisions about the services to be provided to the user.' [3]

- Sitting services which provide someone to sit with the disabled person whilst the carer has time to her/himself are provided by social services and some voluntary organisations.

The most common are those run by Crossroads Care Attendant Schemes, whose phone numbers are listed in Thompson's Directory.

- Benefits which disabled people and carers may be entitled to include:
  ~Attendance Allowance
  ~Disability Living Allowance
  ~Invalid Care Allowance

Most benefits are paid by the Benefits Agency, formerly the DHSS. Some are administered locally, others at central offices.

Eligibility for benefits, and the effects that receiving these particular benefits may have on other benefits and pension is complicated. Most people will need individual advice, and this can be obtained from:

~ Citizens Advice Bureaux (CABs)
~ Independent advice centres
~ Welfare Rights units
~ Disablement associations
~ Age Concern
~ Support agencies such as the Stroke Association

(See Section 6: Some Useful Addresses.)

The Benefits Agency has a Freephone number for disabled people and their carers: 0800 882200 in England, Scotland and Wales: 0800 220674 in Northern Ireland (see page 139)

- Council tax: Carers and disabled people may be entitled to reductions in council tax if:
  - ~ The carer is not included in the number of residents in the household
  - ~ The band value of the property has been lowered because adaptations have been made to the building to accommodate a disabled person.

FURTHER INFORMATION:

- ~ Local Council Tax Office
- ~ Carers' National Association

- Carers' support groups can help to break feelings of isolation by providing the opportunity for carers to talk to others in a similar position.

There are carers' support groups in most parts of the country. The voluntary organisations involved have carers' workers who support carers and help them to access the services they need. These organisations are listed in Thompson's Directory or in the Business section of the phone book under the names of the associations, for example: Stroke Association.

Carers' National Association will also provide details of carers' support organisations. (See Section 6: Some Useful Addresses.)

REFERENCES

1. OPCS Monitor SS92/2 (1992) *General Household Survey: Carers in 1990*. OPCS, London.
2. Ibid
3. Carers (Recognition Services) Act (1995). HMSO, London.

4. *Professional roles in continuing care*

CONTENTS

The general practitioner

Almost everyone in the UK is registered with a general practitioner who is responsible for providing health care on a continuing basis. However it is surprisingly difficult to define this role in a way which is acceptable to all general practitioners because of the way in which general practice has changed over the past 25 years.

In the early days of the Health Service it was generally agreed that the role of general practitioners consisted of making initial or suspected diagnoses and providing or arranging subsequent investigations or treatment.

For many practitioners this still constitutes their major role. However during the past 25 years, in the course of defining a specific role for general practice, other practitioners have accepted that they provide personal primary and continuing medical care to individuals and families. Their diagnoses are therefore composed in physical, psychological and social terms.

Individual practitioners today vary in the extent to which they consider it their responsibility to provide these other aspects of care in addition to the treatment of the disease itself. However whether ongoing review of someone with a chronic incurable condition occurs in general practice or in hospital outpatients, the following list indicates major aspects for a doctor's enquiry:

- Is the diagnosis correct? Have other diagnoses arisen since the last review? Does this person need referral?
- Are the symptoms well controlled?
- Is the treatment appropriate? Should other professions be involved?

- Is the medication appropriate - i.e. effective and without side effects?
- Would this person benefit from instruction in self-help? Is instruction in preventive measures indicated?
- Who are the family/carers?
- What are their roles, problems and needs?
- Does this review cover physical, psychological, emotional and social aspects? If not, to whom should the person be referred?
- Would it be more appropriate for this review to take place in hospital or general practice? Which would the patient prefer?
- Have the patient's views on his/her management and problems been sought?
- Who is the most appropriate person to manage this patient's care?

For optimal care of people with incurable neurological disease and their family/carers, the questions posed above need to be addressed. A broad review is needed, and in many cases the GP will be the most appropriate professional to take the central role in the management of care. This issue is

discussed further in Section 5 of this compendium: Managing Continuing Care.

The nurse

People with neurological disorders often have the most complex health needs encountered by nurses within any care setting. Nurses working with these patients therefore require highly specialised understanding and skills to meet their particular needs.

Skilled, experienced and knowledgeable nurses working with patients who have neurological disorders can provide care which ensures therapeutic effectiveness and quality of life.

Cost effective nursing care saves resources in the longer term. The outcome following nurse intervention may, however, be difficult to measure in terms that are of value to those who hold budgets. It is often difficult to quantify the positive difference qualified nurses make, as so much of what nurses achieve is invisible to health care managers.

High quality nursing is certainly felt and valued by patients, especially those with complex problems. Ill people who are well-dressed and comfortable, able to maintain privacy, dignity and their optimal level of health and independence have received quality nursing care.

The difficulty in evaluating this is due to the fact that nursing is more than a series of separate and identifiable tasks. Many of the subtle nursing activities cannot be readily recognised by the tools commonly used for measurement. Activity analysis categories may record the nurse as washing a patient but they do not record that the nurse is also assessing how the patient is moving or the condition and integrity of the skin. In the process of giving care a nurse will also be talking and listening to the patient, picking up problems such as depression or constipation.

Nurses build up a therapeutic relationship that can make the difference between whether an individual enjoys life or gives up. They have the skills to motivate and empower individuals to maintain their optimal independence. Their role is complementary to that of other health care professionals and pivotal in multi-professional working which is of such importance within neurological disease management.

Qualified nurses have the skills and ability to:

- Recognise the signs and symptoms and subtle changes occurring within an individual which may suggest deterioration
- Prevent complications, deterioration and loss of function
- Use their special skills of rehabilitative nursing in promoting and maintaining independence and functioning capacity
- Set realistic goals with the patients and their families: nurses understand the importance of focusing on abilities rather than deficits to enhance motivation
- Develop expertise in multi-professional working both in health and social care; the nurse can act as a key networker in many situations and maintain continuity of therapeutic support in the absence of other professionals
- Provide up-to-date knowledge of support services which can help to maintain the patient in the community and prevent admission into hospital
- Understand mental changes patients may develop in some neurological disorders and the importance of assessing the needs these changes may bring
- Involve, teach and support the carers of those with neurological disorders so that they can enjoy quality of life within their caring role

Nurses have a key role to play in the management of neurological disorders: assessing needs, supporting individuals and their carers and anticipating the care required. They are often instrumental in setting up support systems for patients and in many cases can act as a key worker to maintain continuity of therapeutic support in the absence of other professionals.

Nurse specialists

Patient treatment and care have become more complex over the last ten years, largely because of modern technology and drug therapy, and the role of the nurse specialist has increased considerably during this time. This has particularly been the case in the field of neurology, where there are now many nurse specialists who work in either acute or community settings, or a combination of the two.

Nurse specialists in neurological disorders may be employed directly by NHS Trusts and community units, by charitable organisations, or by the commercial sector.

Their role involves advising GPs, generalist nurses, patients and carers on treatment and care options, and they have a range of duties including:

- Disease management
- Health promotion and maintenance of health
- Counselling
- Consumer education
- Professional education

Some nurse specialists are directly involved in education, research and audit and have little, if any, direct contact with patients. Examples of nurse specialists include:

- Continence nurse specialists
- Parkinson's disease nurse specialists
- Epilepsy nurse specialists
- Multiple sclerosis nurse specialists

This list is not exhaustive. To find out if there is a disease specific nurse specialist in your area you can contact your local hospital or the relevant charitable association for that specific disease, for example, the Parkinson's Disease Society. The Continence Foundation holds a register of Continence Nurse Specialists. The addresses of these organisations can be found in Section 6 of this compendium.

Failing this, contact the Information Officer, Royal College of Nursing, 20 Cavendish Square, London WIM OAB. Tel: 0171 409 3333.

FURTHER READING

Atkin, K., Twigg J. (1993) Nurses effectiveness in supporting carers. *Nursing Standard,* **7:7:4,** 38 - 39.

Jones, A. (1995) Utilising Peplau's Psychodynamic Theory for Stroke Patient Care. *The Journal of Clinical Nursing,* **4:1,** 49 - 54.

O'Brien, J., Austin, M., Sethi, P., O'Boyle, P. (1991) Urinary Incontinence: Prevalence. Need for Treatment and Effectiveness of Intervention by Nurse. *British Medical Journal,* **303,** 1308 - 1311.

Royal College of Nursing (1992) *The Value of Nursing.* RCN, London.

Thomas, S. (1995) Managing Parkinson's Disease. *Community Outlook*, **4:6,** 15 - 20.

The health visitor

Health visitors are registered nurses who have undertaken further post-registration training in order to qualify and register as health visitors with the UKCC which is the nurses', midwives' and health visitors' statutory body. That training includes psychology, sociology and social policy as well as public health.

Health visitors work in the community alongside general practitioners. They visit clients in their homes or other community settings and can add valuable skills to those of the primary health care team.

The main focus of their work is health promotion and primary prevention. However, the widely-held belief that health visitors work only with mothers and young children is incorrect. Health visitors use their many and varied skills to work with individuals of all ages, their families and the communities within which they live. There are also specialist health visitors in specific fields who work with the elderly, the homeless, and children and families with special needs.

Although they are nurses, health visitors do not perform typical nursing roles. However, they do have a caring role as well which can encompass physical, mental, psychological or social continuing care, and involves:

- Listening to and considering the nature of problems
- Guiding and supporting patients and their family and carers in understanding and coming to terms with their condition
- Identifying need and offering information and advice best suited to the health requirements, in the broadest sense, of the individual, the carer and family

Health visitors are generally employed by NHS Community Care Trusts or health authorities. Many now work with GPs as part of primary health care teams. Although they work mainly in the community, health visitors also have close and easily accessible links with acute units (hospitals), other community units, and other services. They are therefore ideally placed to explain networks and the working of these other services to patients and their carers.

In working with people with neurological disorders, health visitors can also work with their families and with the communities in which they live to promote awareness and campaign for adequate facilities.

People with neurological disorders often find it comforting or reassuring to know the health visitor is a nurse, but that she also has wide knowledge in other fields of caring. The health visitor can offer holistic and continuing care to help meet the needs of the individual physically, psychologically, mentally and socially.

USEFUL ADDRESS

Health Visitors' Association
50 Southwark Street
London SE1
Tel: 0171 717 4000

Offers general information about the role of health visitors, and specific information about special interest groups within the profession.

Psychological support professionals

The need for psychological and emotional support for those suffering from neurological disorders, and for their carers, has been highlighted throughout the earlier sections of this compendium. Increasing recognition of the need for psychological support has led to the evolution of a number of different models of access to these services. The precise model depends on local conditions and resources.

In areas served by a community mental health team (CMHT) access is often made through a referral, generally by the GP, to an appropriate member of the team. An individual key worker will then be allocated to the patient. In services where there is no CMHT, referral can generally be made directly through the individual professional attached to the patient's care team or hospital.

The choice of appropriate support will depend on the range of services available locally, but is likely to come from one of the following professions:

- Community psychiatric nurse
- Clinical psychologists
- Counselling psychologists/counsellors

THE COMMUNITY PSYCHIATRIC NURSE

Community psychiatric nurses (CPNs), sometimes known as community mental health nurses, are qualified nurses who use their mental nursing skills working with people in their own homes.

Most are still employed and based within mental health services, forming part of CMHT where they work with psychiatrists, psychologists, social workers and occupational therapists. However they are increasingly being employed by other agencies such as GP fundholding practices, social services departments, independent and voluntary sector organisations.

In GP practices the CPN acts as a formal link. Members of the primary care team can discuss potential referrals and seek support, supervision and advice on management. This may obviate the need for formal referral. Where referral is made, the CPN will assess and, if appropriate, accept the patient for treatment.

When working with people with neurological disorders the CPN's roles include that of: consultant, clinician, therapist, assessor, educator and manager.[1] CPNs can help both patient and family to understand what is happening: the nature of the disorder, its progress, effects and treatment. In some cases they may be the key person in the management of a patient's care (see Section 5: Managing Continuing Care).

For example, in the case of a person with Alzheimer's disease the CPN's role could involve:

- Assessing the person's behaviour
- Planning a routine or schedule with the patient and family which can be easily followed
- Using stress management techniques and training to help the carer as the condition progresses
- Using reminiscence therapy to help the patient overcome frustrations over the loss of short term memory and exercise his or her brain function
- Helping develop strategies with the family to deal with concerns over wandering and safety in the home
- Introducing family and carer to self-support groups - in some cases running their meetings

Clinical psychologists

Clinical psychologists apply psychological theory and practice to a broad range of mental, physical and emotional problems. They use their skills in helping patients to clarify their problems, and draw on psychological knowledge and theory to assess their needs, recommend interventions and evaluate outcomes.

Clinical psychologists work with different groups including children, young people and families, older people, people with learning disabilities, people with physical disabilities and those with neurological conditions, dealing with emotional, addiction and habit problems, psychosocial difficulties, social and interpersonal difficulties, psychosomatic and medical illnesses, and challenging behaviour.

There is now a small, but growing number of clinical psychologists who specialise in neuropsychology. They bring a unique perspective to the assessment of neuropsychological impairment and its relationship to behaviour and consider this in the light of career and educational background together with emotional difficulties such as depression and anxiety.

Counselling psychologists/counsellors also work with people with a variety of problems and needs, for example, those suffering bereavements and relationship problems, or carers, helping them adjust to changes in the person for whom they are caring.

Involving psychologists in the care of people with neurological disorders can result in the following improvements in the care of the individual, and support for their carer:

- A more comprehensive assessment of acute neurological conditions, leading to greater efficiency in diagnosis
- Greater understanding of impairments caused by the disease, resulting in a more appropriate treatment and management plan

- Teaching new skills and strategies to circumvent intellectual/cognitive impairment
- Use of appropriate techniques to manage (if treatment is not practical) difficult behaviour, resulting in reduced stress to the individual, the carers and to health and education professionals
- Reduction in the frequency or severity of problem behaviours, such as aggression, violence or sexual disinhibition, which can limit the duration of hospital admission or readmission and can potentially reduce the frequency of outpatient referrals to specialist units by early intervention and appropriate management
- Advice to carers on management strategies, and how to reduce their own stress can improve confidence in their ability to cope, which may result in early discharge of the patient from hospital
- Improvements in mental health and reduction in symptoms of depression and anxiety in the client, the carer and family
- Supporting and liaising with employees and teachers to enable a return to work or to education at a more appropriate stage
- Reduced reliance on medication to suppress problem behaviour

Clinical psychologists can support the primary health care team in a number of ways. They can help in:

- Clarifying queries over diagnosis
- Advising on practical issues such as the ability to live independently or to return to work or education
- Assisting in the formulation of a management/treatment plan set at an appropriate level

Most Health Trusts have departments of clinical psychology, some have departments of clinical and counselling psychology.

Counselling psychologists/counsellors

Counselling also has a role in helping patients and their family/carers to understand and deal with complex and confusing emotional responses to their condition. Counselling psychologists/counsellors can help in a variety of ways - psychodynamically, systemically and interpersonally by:

- Helping the person work through feelings of loss, including loss of identity, of role, of physical well-being, of sexual functioning
- Enabling the person to develop insight into his/her own and other people's complex responses
- Enabling couples and families to come to terms with difficult and unacceptable feelings and to communicate more openly and confidently with respect to these
- Facilitating emotional and interpersonal adjustment to a new sense of self

This type of psychological input, which often takes place over a longer period, enables people to live more independent and happy lives, both personally and interpersonally.

The choice as to which is the most appropriate type of psychological support depends on the individual needs of the patient and the carer, and these should be carefully assessed before any such decision is made by the person managing that patient's care.

References

1. Carr, P. J., et al (1980) *Community Psychiatric Nursing*. Churchill Livingstone, London.

Further reading

DoH (1994) *Working in Partnership: The Report of the Mental Health Nursing Review*. Department of Health, London.

Useful addresses

Community Psychiatric Nurses' Association
'Cais Meyn'
Grove Lane
Hinton
Chippenham SN14 8HF
Tel: 0117 937 3365 Fax: 0117 937 4892
Email: 101632.1366@compuserve.com

British Psychological Society
St Andrew's House
48 Princess Road East
Leicester LE1 7DR
Tel: 0116 254 9568

Also has specialist groups in clinical psychology, counselling psychology and neuropsychology.

British Association for Counselling
Tel: 01788 578328

The social services department

Social services department staff have a key role to play in the care of people with neurological disorders who want to remain at home. Although the structure of social services departments varies widely from one part of the country to another, their responsibilities under the National Health Service and Community Care Act, 1990, and other legislation, are the same.

'Care management is the process of tailoring services to individual needs' [1]

In some departments, social workers work as care managers and their key functions are to assess needs and organise care packages. In others, the focus is more on the traditional role of offering support to disabled people and their families. Social workers can provide, or open the door to many different services, enabling people to live in their own homes for as long as possible, with dignity and a reasonable quality of life. When this is no longer possible, social workers can arrange appropriate residential or nursing care.

The NHS Community Care Act 1990 (section 47) has given the local authority 'lead responsibility' for assessment and care management of community care services and one of the key objectives for service delivery is to:

'make proper assessment of need and good case management the cornerstone of high quality care' [2]

Social workers may be employed either in the hospital setting, where they should be involved in making sure that services are organised before a patient is discharged home, or in the community where they have responsibilities under various pieces of legislation for the following:

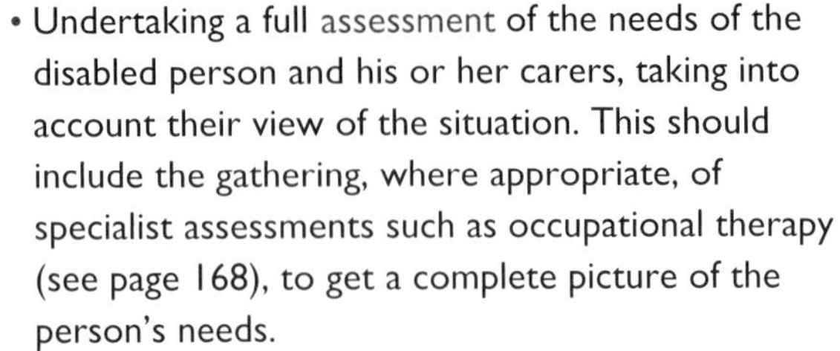

- Undertaking a full assessment of the needs of the disabled person and his or her carers, taking into account their view of the situation. This should include the gathering, where appropriate, of specialist assessments such as occupational therapy (see page 168), to get a complete picture of the person's needs.

- Development of a care package - the complete range of assistance necessary from Health and Social Services to meet the identified needs of the patient/client. The package might simply involve the provision of a single service, or it might be much more complex and include a range of services, such as mobile meals, day care, respite care, practical and personal assistance, specialist equipment and/or adaptations to the home, nursing services, speech and/or physiotherapy and chiropody.
- Co-ordination of service provision, and liaison with other professionals involved, including arranging any case conferences or meetings which may be necessary.
- Monitoring to ensure that services are provided and continue to be appropriate.
- Regular review of the Care Plan, making sure that needs are still being met.
- Advocacy for the service user, if appropriate. Sometimes an independent advocate, perhaps from a voluntary organisation, is more appropriate.
- Counselling in so far as it relates to the above functions. It may be appropriate to obtain specialist counselling from a voluntary sector agency such as a bereavement service or neurological charity, or from a mental health professional (see page 157).

- General advice about welfare benefits to ensure that people are receiving their full entitlements (see page 136, Section 3: Social Difficulties).

Many patients with neurological illness access continuing care through social services, rather than health care services, and it is important that effective links exist between the two. This is discussed further in Section 5: Managing Continuing Care.

References

1. *Care Management and Assessment: Summary of Practice Guidance.* (1991) Department of Health Social Services Inspectorate, HMSO, London.

2. *Caring for people: Community Care in the next Decade and Beyond, Key objectives for service delivery* (1989) HMSO, London.

PROFESSIONAL ROLES 4

The physiotherapist

Chartered physiotherapists aim to help each individual to re-establish a role within his or her environment. For patients with neurological disorders they assist in obtaining optimal function and alleviating discomfort, while working towards agreed goals.

The physiotherapist assesses the patient and, together with the person and the carer, if appropriate, devises a tailor-made programme to meet the individual's needs. The outcomes of this programme are continuously monitored and changed as the person's state alters. Those with progressive conditions are helped to maintain as much mobility as possible for as long as possible, perhaps with the help of aids, such as wheelchairs or walking frames.

The physiotherapy treatment of patients with neurological problems requires advanced education not only in anatomy and physiology, but also in normal and abnormal movement patterns. The skill required in the therapeutic handling of patients with neurological deficit is complex and takes time to acquire. Neurology is a speciality within physiotherapy for which staff undergo post-graduate training. A senior neurological physiotherapist will normally have been qualified for at least five years, with three years in the neurological field, and have undertaken relevant courses.

Chartered physiotherapists in neurology:

- Help optimise patients' physical function and comfort.
- Assess and diagnose each patient from a physiotherapeutic point of view. This includes the patient's past and current medical history, his/her physical, psychological and social needs, quality of movement, abilities and functional independence.

- Devise a physiotherapy management programme and goals agreed with the patient and carer, taking account of the patient's wishes to establish or maintain a role within his/her own environment.
- Continue to monitor the patient's state, changing and adapting the goals and programme as necessary.
- Ensure rehabilitation or maintenance programmes are understood and complemented by all members of the health care team.
- Liaise with the patient's carers and relatives to ensure that they can help the patient to achieve his/her maximum potential.
- Ensure that the patient and carers are aware of relevant support groups and charities.
- When discharging from physiotherapy, ensure that each patient has a planned programme to follow.

Chartered physiotherapists have a pivotal role in the rehabilitation or maintenance of people with neurological problems. They help the patient to make the most of any potential for recovery or to maintain, for as long as possible, their mobility and dignity.

FURTHER READING

Standards of Physiotherapy Practice in Neurology (1995) The Chartered Society of Physiotherapy.

Recommendations for Physiotherapy Practice and Service Development in Neurology (1995) The Chartered Society of Physiotherapy.

References for the efficacy of physiotherapy in the treatment of individual neurological conditions are available from:

Research Development Officer
Chartered Society of Physiotherapy
14 Bedford Row
London WC1R 4ED

The occupational therapist

Occupational therapists aim to assist individuals to develop and maintain their capacity to perform, at a level satisfying to themselves and others, the tasks and roles essential to productive living and optimal functioning within their own environment.

The occupational therapist assesses the person's ability to perform effectively self-care, productivity and leisure tasks, and can implement a programme to enable him or her to learn or relearn specific activities, develop skills, adapt behaviour or to adjust the environment to meet specific needs.

The occupational therapist functions in the following ways:

- Analysing with the client those activities of daily life which are most important and useful to him or her
- Analysing the skills needed to perform specific activities
- Helping clients to organise and balance the sequence of activity within their daily routine
- Suggesting alternative or adaptive ways of carrying out activities
- Providing resources for practising and trying out different ways of performing activities
- Advising on or providing specialised equipment to assist in the performance of daily activities

Outcomes for the clients should include:

- The achievement of optimal functioning within their own environment
- Successful adaptation and adjustment to their changed/changing circumstances
- Autonomy or functional independence - where self-management is the key

- An increased sense of accomplishment, satisfaction and control over their lives
- An improved level of physical and mental health and sense of well-being
- An increased sense of dignity and self worth through the knowledge that ability, not disability is important to their quality of life

Occupational therapists working with people with neurological disorders may work either for the community health service as part of the primary health care team, or for the local authority in social services.

Occupational therapists employed in social services departments by the local authority undertake full functional assessments of those who have severe physical disabilities and their families. The aim is to maximise people's independence, improve their quality of life and support carers.

They primarily deal with:

- Reinforcing and supporting the rehabilitation programme which started in hospital
- Providing equipment and minor adaptations to the home
- Drawing up specifications, where major alterations to the home are necessary in order that the person may live safely at home (for example, the installation of a stair lift or a downstairs lavatory or bathroom)
- Making recommendations for financial assistance under the various grants which are available, and liaising with the Environmental Health Departments who usually administer the grants, and architects
- Advising on all issues concerning the safe moving and lifting of disabled people
- Providing advice and recommendations on transport issues, for example, Disabled Parking bays outside the person's home, Orange Badges, Disabled Driving issues and wheelchair mobility

Access to occupational therapy services will vary from area to area, depending on what resources are available, and how they are organised. Although it is becoming more common for GPs to refer patients to occupational therapy via the primary health care team, the most usual approach is still via social services (see Section 5: Managing Continuing Care).

Further reading

Reed, K., Sanderson, S. (1985) *Concepts of Occupational Therapy*. Williams and Wilkins, London.

Useful address

Disability Information and Study Centre (DISC)
The College of Occupational Therapists
6-8 Marshalsea Road
London SE1 1HL
Tel: 0171 357 6480

The speech and language therapist

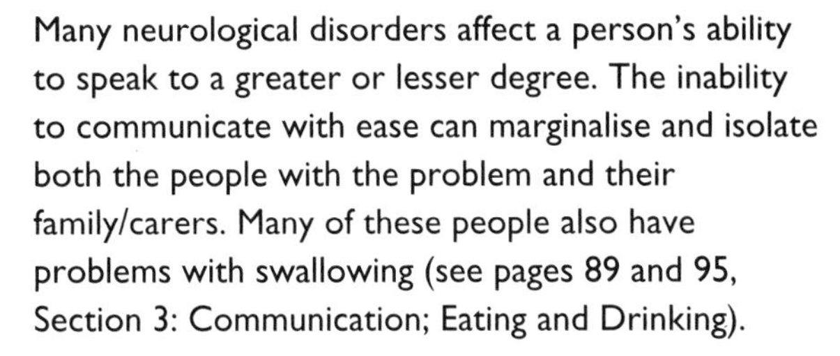

Many neurological disorders affect a person's ability to speak to a greater or lesser degree. The inability to communicate with ease can marginalise and isolate both the people with the problem and their family/carers. Many of these people also have problems with swallowing (see pages 89 and 95, Section 3: Communication; Eating and Drinking).

Speech and language therapists have now broadened their remit to assist in the management of dysphagia as well dysarthria, dysphasia and other communication impairments.

A registered speech and language therapist has the knowledge and skills to help:

- People who have difficulties in communicating in any way at any stage, including those whose ability to communicate is deteriorating
- The family/carers who are also affected by the communication problems, because they cannot understand the sufferer and because of the emotional stress this creates for all concerned
- People who have swallowing difficulties

Early assessment by a speech and language therapist is vital, as the therapist can help to maintain the level of communication, either verbally or if necessary with the use of communication aids.

Some GPs feel that it may waste the resources of a speech and language therapist to refer people whose condition is deteriorating. This is not so. Speech and language therapists are trained to both assess and treat people with communication disorders ranging from mild to severe impairment. Where direct therapy may not be appropriate, much can still be done to alleviate stress for those with the disorder and their family/carers.

Whilst the advantages of such work are not shown easily by traditional research methodology, there is a growing body of research to support intervention, which includes a list of efficacy studies for dysphasia which is available from Action for Dysphasic Adults (see page 194, Section 6: Some Useful Addresses).

Research indicates that speech and language therapy has a positive role to play in managing problems arising in progressive neurological diseases.

In order to ensure that the speech and language therapist is appropriately qualified and adheres to the professional standards of practice, the GP should check that the therapist is registered by contacting the Royal College of Speech and Language Therapists.

Speech and language therapists work in a variety of settings:

- Hospitals
- Community centres
- Nursing homes
- The patients' homes

Further reading

Enderby, P., Emerson, J. (1995) *Does Speech and Language Therapy Work?* Whurr Publications, London.

Useful addresses

Information on how to contact a speech and language therapist in your area is available from:

The Royal College of Speech and Language Therapists
7 Bath Place
Rivington Street
London EC2A 3DR
Tel: 0171 613 3855

5. Managing continuing care

Contents

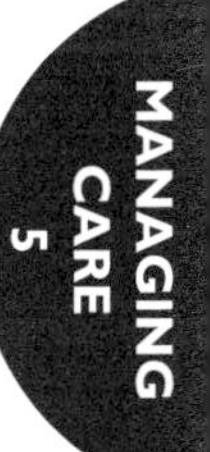

Managing continuing care

People with neurological disorders will obtain continuing care through one of three routes:

- Their GP
- On discharge from hospital
- The social services

Whatever their condition, and wherever they live, these people will be receiving care against a background of continuing change in health and social services, resulting in wide variations in what is available to them from one area to another. These variations will in turn influence the way an individual's care is managed thereafter, and the role of the GP in that management.

The aim of this section is illustrate that whatever the local conditions, there are some important general principles relating to the management of continuing care which will apply regardless of local and political issues. These principles place the patient and carer at the centre of the process, and view the various services discussed in Section 4 of this compendium as providing support which meets their individual needs.

Surveys of these patients and their family carers have shown that their prime needs are:

- An accurate diagnosis and the best treatment
- Appropriate information
- To be listened to and their difficulties understood
- Support through a difficult time

There are two case studies in this section, written by a GP to illustrate some of the ways in which the GP can be involved in meeting these needs. These scenarios are used to illustrate the principles of managing continuing care, and they are followed by discussion which explores how these principles may apply in the context of variations in local services.

Planning continuing care

The way continuing care is managed will be governed to a large extent by the resources available within the area and how easily they can be accessed. Provision of health services varies widely throughout the country. The resources available in one place may not be available in another. Access to a particular service or to key people may be through different channels in different areas.

Relations between social and health services and between social services and general practices also vary.

Figure 1 on the next page shows how an understanding of the roles of different professionals (see Section 4) can lead to more informed decision-making about how to meet the needs of individual patients and their carers. Knowledge about who does what and how well within the existing constraints will strongly influence decisions about when and where continuing care should be provided and who should provide it.

It is vital, where effective continuing care involves many professionals, sometimes at the same time, sometimes consecutively, to have one person who adopts a co-ordinating or key role in managing that care. In many cases, the GP will be the most appropriate person, either acting alone or in conjunction with social services, to fulfil that role.

As the balance of care shifts from the hospital to the community sector, it is increasingly important to devise appropriate and effective shared care

Figure 1 Assessment of the ongoing needs of patients and family carers

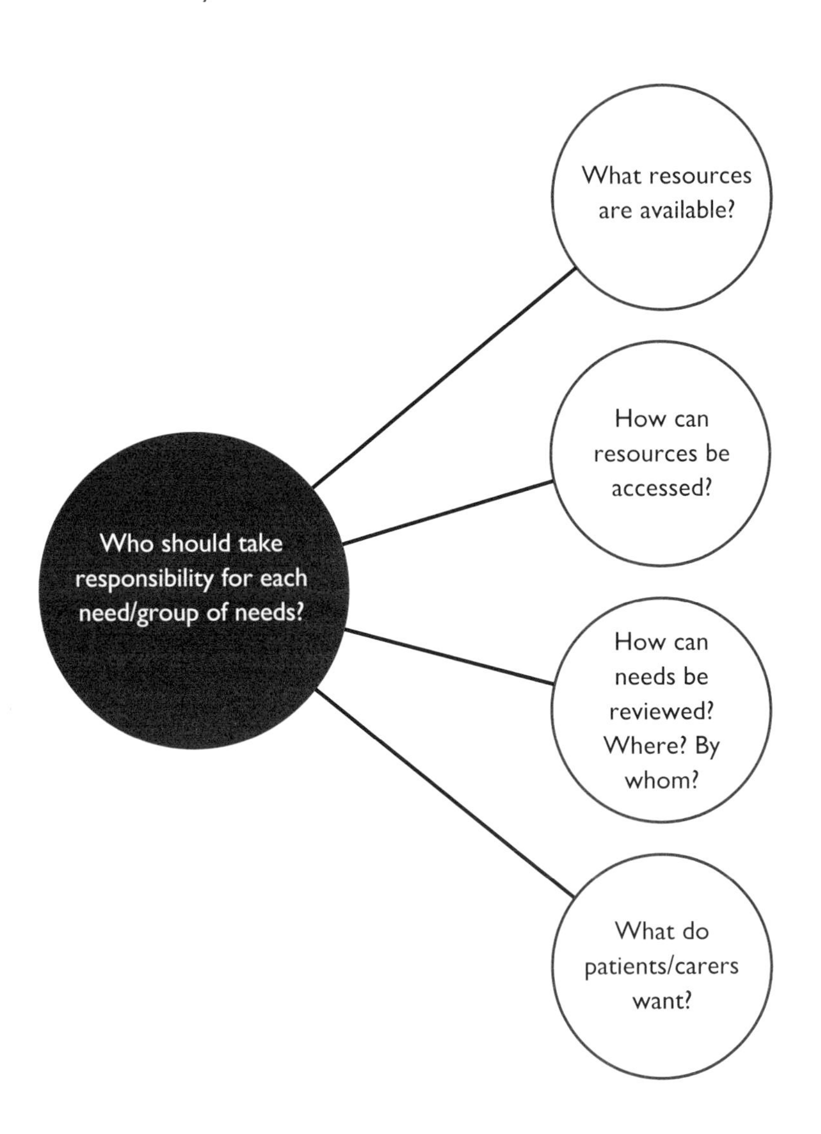

protocols, with agreed criteria for good care. The details of such protocols will depend on the particular condition or disease involved, but the principles underpinning the protocols are those identified by the patients and their carers:

- Accurate diagnosis and best treatment
- Appropriate information
- To be listened to and their difficulties understood
- Appropriate support through difficult times

Figure 2 on the next page shows how a protocol for a review procedure could be developed. Similar questions can be asked before the introduction of any new activity to ensure that all parties involved are well-informed and in agreement.

When new activities involving more than one person are introduced in any organisation or situation, success depends on general agreement on:

- Whether the activity is worth doing
- The desired outcome
- What should be done to achieve it
- Who should do it

The initiative is most likely to succeed if reviews of method and outcome are built into the plan (see figure 2).

Multidisciplinary care teams are essential but cannot work efficiently without good communication.

Once the key people have been identified, and a protocol for shared care developed, how best can we make use of the professionals selected for the maximum benefit of patient and carer? The following is a checklist of questions which can aid decisions about the most appropriate course to take in the management of neurological disorders.

Figure 2 Development of a protocol for a review procedure

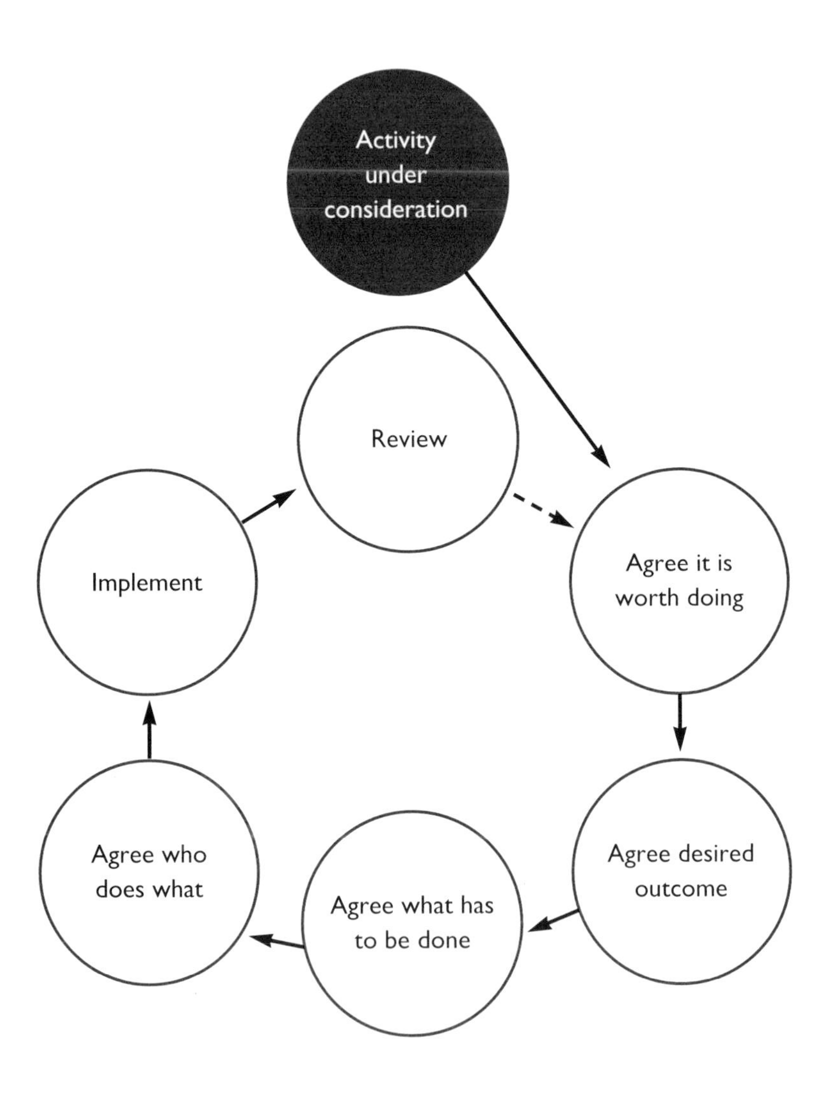

Primary care

Primary care, and often the GP, is the first point of contact for most patients. In considering the initial management and provisional diagnosis:

- Where is it most appropriate for this person to receive care - primary care or secondary care?
- Who is the most appropriate professional to deal with it (e.g. in primary care, is it the GP, or might someone else be more appropriate)?
- When to refer? (Can it ever be too soon or too late?)
- Which neurologist has a particular expertise/interest in the condition?
- Why is referral taking place?
- What resources are available in your locality?
- What is the role of the primary health care team?
- How can access to the relevant key people be made?

Secondary care

- Why involve secondary care?
- When should secondary care be involved?
- Who is the relevant specialist for this patient (e.g. neurologist, gerontologist, liaison nurse)?
- What is good shared care? Are there agreed protocols?
- Initial support
- What are the plans for follow-up once the diagnosis has been given to the patient?
- Who is involved? For example: the specialist/GP/nurse/physiotherapist?
- What resources are available?
- What has the patient been told in relation to his/her diagnosis and management?

The process of managing continuing care

The key to successful management of continuing care lies in two factors:

- Understanding of the required outcomes for patient and carer
- Knowledge of the resources available in the locality and how they are organised

These can be brought together using a needs-based assessment within the context of local provision, using the following guidelines:

Assessment:
~ Why assess this patient?
~ When should the assessment/s be made?
~ Who should do it?
~ How might it be carried out?

Planning:
~ Who should be involved?
~ What resources are available for patient and carer?
~ How can we keep it relevant to their needs?

Implementation: Assessment and planning will be a waste of time if implementation does not take place and quickly.
~ Who should be responsible for the implementation of care?
~ When should it begin?
~ How should it be implemented?

Evaluation: Continuing care needs to be relevant for the individual patient and carer and they need to be brought centre stage in the evaluation process.
~ Who should be involved?
~ When should evaluation take place?
~ How should care and services be evaluated?

Figure 3 shows how the various different agencies might be combined in the continuing care of a patient with Parkinson's disease. This figure is based on a real model currently in use in a GP practice. The diagram is supplied to patients and their carers with a list of all the relevant local addresses on the back.

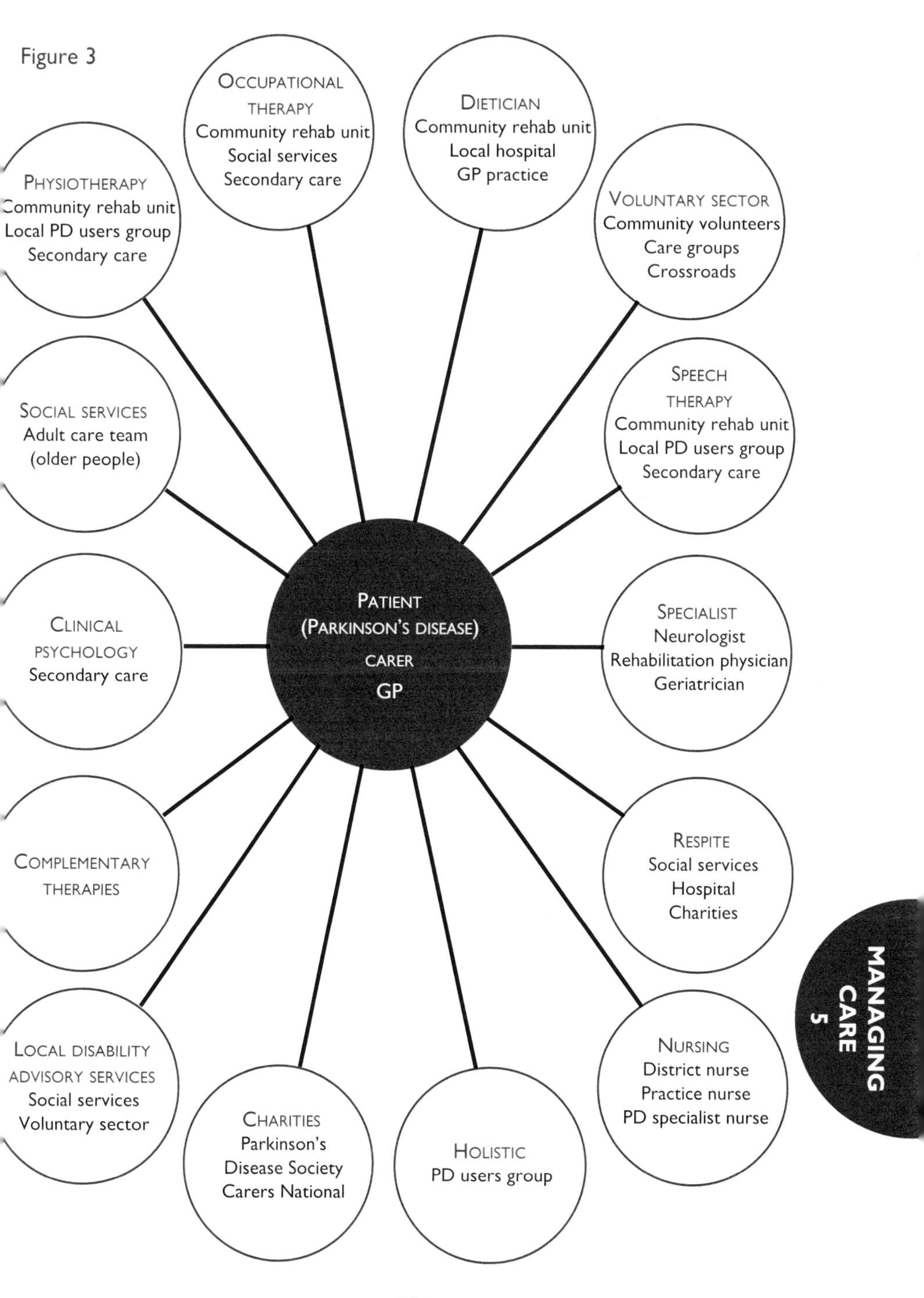
Figure 3
Occupational therapy
Community rehab unit
Social services
Secondary care
Dietician
Community rehab unit
Local hospital
GP practice
Physiotherapy
Community rehab unit
Local PD users group
Secondary care
Voluntary sector
Community volunteers
Care groups
Crossroads
Social services
Adult care team
(older people)
Speech therapy
Community rehab unit
Local PD users group
Secondary care
Patient
(Parkinson's disease)
carer
GP
Clinical psychology
Secondary care
Specialist
Neurologist
Rehabilitation physician
Geriatrician
Complementary therapies
Respite
Social services
Hospital
Charities
Local disability advisory services
Social services
Voluntary sector
Charities
Parkinson's
Disease Society
Carers National
Holistic
PD users group
Nursing
District nurse
Practice nurse
PD specialist nurse
MANAGING CARE
5

CASE STUDIES

The following two case studies illustrate:

- How the issues outlined in this section of the compendium might work in practice
- The GP's involvement in the initial management and continuing care of two patients with contrasting sets of problems

They are not, of course, intended to be prescriptive, and the discussion which follows highlights some of the many ways in which the scenarios could have varied, and some of the different options which might have been chosen in their management.

Case I David

David is 38. He is an accountant who lives with his girlfriend, Maggie. They have no children.

David presents to his GP with signs and symptoms which strongly support a diagnosis of multiple sclerosis.

- The GP decides that David needs an early specialist opinion, and refers him to a consultant neurologist who confirms the diagnosis and considers the best options for managing his condition.
- The neurologist then informs the GP of his recommendations, including: who else has knowledge of the diagnosis; plans for follow-up, for example, to monitor David for depression following the confirmation of the diagnosis; what rehabilitation needs have been advised; what further investigations are planned; what treatment options have been discussed.
- Soon after this, the GP arranges to see David and Maggie to explore their health beliefs and understanding of multiple sclerosis, and to try to identify the nature of the support they are likely to

need. He tries to be aware of functional as well as clinical criteria in assessing these immediate and future needs.

- At this stage the GP's aim is to develop a good relationship with David and Maggie, and to be seen as someone who is a professional family friend to support them through a difficult time.
- David's main problem is mobility, and the GP, in consultation with the neurologist, refers him to the local rehabilitation unit for physiotherapy and occupational therapy. The unit provides feedback to the GP on David's progress approximately every three months. He also attends a local MS therapy centre, but at this stage he chooses not to be involved with the MS Society.
- David does not want social services involved at this stage either. His employers, a firm of accountants, are very supportive regarding any necessary absence from work, and he has personal health insurance if he is absent for any length of time. Maggie is a great support and seems to be coping.
- Although Maggie is not a patient of the practice, David's GP is aware of the carer's strain index, and suggests that she sees her own GP if necessary. She does not at this stage wish to be involved with Carers' National Association.
- David is keen on self-help, the options for complementary therapies, diet, and holistic aspects of care. He finds *MS - the self-help guide* by Judy Graham[1] especially helpful.
- David continues under periodic review by the neurologist (approximately six-monthly). There is a unit in the region which evaluates people for beta interferon, and although David does not fully fulfil the criteria for giving beta interferon, the neurologist keeps this particular management option under review.

- David had a major relapse lasting 3 months, during which he was virtually housebound, although he remained self-sufficient, and his condition did not require that Maggie give up work to care for him. The issues for work, driving and the physical and emotional consequences were explored during more regular contact with his GP. During this period, the GP continued with his aim of being an informed professional family friend without medicalising everything.

Discussion This case illustrates some of the issues relating to the role of the GP in managing the care of a patient in the early stages of a neurological disease.

David's care involved the following elements:

- Self-help
- The GP
- The local community health services
- Technical and specialist support from the consultant neurologist

In this scenario the neurologist and the GP had good knowledge of the local care options, and there was effective co-ordination between the different elements. The GP was the key to the success of the management and support system, and was well-informed by the various parties involved in David's care. David himself was well-educated and self-aware, and took steps to inform himself of the care and support options available to him. The GP was proactive in initiating contact where he felt it was appropriate, even though his role in actually providing 'medical' care was limited at this stage in David's illness.

In this particular case, the GP practice had a system for collecting data about the patient's care which was held by David so that anyone involved in his care could see what else was involved. The situation could have been further improved by the development of a shared care protocol and agreed criteria for good practice in relation to people with MS.

There are, of course, several ways in which the situation described here could be varied to place different demands on the role of the GP. For example, he might have had to actively seek out the information about the original consultation with the neurologist, and find out for himself about the options which had been considered. This would have been essential for him to play the co-ordinating role effectively.

The patient may have been less well-informed than David, and the GP would have had a greater role in seeking out and supplying information about the condition, the treatment options (including self-help) and the support available. He might, too, have found himself in the position where his assessment of the situation, and the carer's ability to cope, suggested that it would be advisable to involve social services in some way at an earlier stage. He would have had to find ways of persuading the patient that this was desirable.

In fact, it is possible that later on in David's care management he will have to do this anyway, if his condition deteriorates and places additional strain on Maggie, his carer.

Case 2 Winifred

Winifred is 76. She has been a widow for two years, and has generally been independent and self-caring during this time. She has no family. She has been known to social services for some years since she was assessed as a carer when her husband had a CVA. She moved locally into sheltered housing 12 months ago when she joined the practice, but she is not particularly well-known by the practice. She

has been referred to her GP by social services because of falls.

- Her GP decides to visit at home with the social worker. This allows him to make not only a clinical but also a functional assessment of Winifred in her relatively new environment. It also gives him the opportunity to develop a relationship with her social worker, and to share in decisions about her future care.
- His assessment reveals symptoms and signs of osteoarthritis, Parkinson's disease and mild depression. He decides that the osteoarthritis and depression are manageable within primary care. Socially she is a little isolated, so arrangements are made to attend a day centre for lunch three days a week, and review of social contact within her sheltered accommodation is discussed with the warden.
- She has quite marked tremor, some rigidity and bradykinesia. The GP decides to refer Winifred to a neurologist who runs a movement disorder clinic. He is aware that misdiagnosis can occur in 25 per cent of cases of Parkinson's disease.
- Parkinson's disease is diagnosed. Winifred is placed on Madopar, and followed up in the clinic six weeks later. She is also seen by the Parkinson's disease liaison nurse, who liaises with the GP. A plan for shared care is agreed with the GP, the neurologist and the various therapy groups, and six-monthly review by the neurologist is agreed as adequate at the moment.
- The GP and the PD liaison nurse outline various support options to Winifred. She decides that she would like to join the local branch of the Parkinson's Disease Society. She also chooses to join a local PD users group where physiotherapy is based on the principles of conductive education

which require Winifred's active participation in reaching achievable goals. Participation in this group reduces her feelings of isolation and helps her motivation and confidence.

- The GP keeps other options for care under review, including speech and language therapy, respite care and nursing care. Winifred occasionally uses the voluntary sector for public transport to the day centre, and she has had an occupational therapy home assessment by social services.
- Winifred's mobility and her mood improve, and she continues for the moment self-caring and moderately independent. Since she has no family, her social and medical care are kept discreetly under review by social services and her GP, who has gradually moved forward to 'jobshare' the role of key worker with social services. He also appreciates the support when required from the neurologist in sharing the management of her Parkinson's disease.

Discussion This case illustrates how health and social services combined to manage the care of a patient with health problems due to ageing and a specific neurological condition.

Again, the GP was proactive in creating a key role which ensured that the various agencies involved in Winifred's care were co-ordinated, and that appropriate information was available when it was needed.

His knowledge of local resources led him to refer Winifred to the neurologist. He might, if such resources had existed locally, have decided to refer her to a consultant geriatrician instead.

The PD liaison nurse is a key figure in Winifred's care, acting as an important link between primary and secondary care in the early stages of care management. Once again, not all areas have someone in this role, and had the PD nurse not been available, then the GP would have assumed this linking role, bridging the gap between hospital and community care.

These two cases illustrate some of the key principles involved in managing continuing care of people with neurological disorders.These principles can be summed up into five areas which provide the key to effective management of continuing care:

---

1 Knowledge of the needs of and services required by patients and their domestic carers is particularly important for health and social service professionals involved in a provider and purchaser role at a time of great change at local and national level.
2 Information for patients and carers, health and social services professionals, should be well co-ordinated and accessible.
3 Communication. Inter-professional barriers have to be broken down and communication between all those responsible for caring for the chronically ill and disabled needs to be excellent.
4 Assessment. General practitioners should be encouraged to use functional rather than clinical criteria for assessing individuals' disabilities.
5 Remember the carer. The family/carer is the key to effective continuing care. Carers' needs should be borne in mind by professionals, and assessed and taken into account as much as those of the patient.

REFERENCE

1. Graham, J. (1992) *Multiple Sclerosis - the self-help guide*. Harper Collins, London.

6. *Some useful addresses*

CONTENTS

The following lists contain the addresses already given in the Factfile, which also gives more details about the services they can offer to professionals, patients and carers. This section also contains addresses of other organisations which can offer support and other services to people with neurological conditions and their carers.

Health support

General health organisations

A patient's first port of call will normally be his or her GP but general information can be obtained from:

Health Information Service
Tel: Freephone 0800 66 55 44

The Freephone Health Information Service provides a helpline where anyone with health concerns can seek information. Callers are automatically routed to the nearest regional health information service.

The helpline is designed to provide information on common diseases and conditions, NHS services, waiting times, local Patient's Charter standards, how to complain about the NHS, and how to maintain good health. The helpline can also provide information on self-help groups and voluntary services in local areas.

Publication *A Practical Guide for Disabled People: where to find information, services and equipment.*

This extremely clear, useful and wide-ranging guide is available free of charge, from Department of Health, PO Box 410, Wetherby LS23 7LN. It is also available from this address as an audio cassette, and in braille.

The following organisations also offer advice and information:

Community Health Councils (CHCs) (see the Business section of the telephone directory) can help with concerns and complaints about NHS services and treatment, including registering with a GP or changing to a new GP. They also have details of local dentists and opticians.

The Association for Community Health Councils has published a leaflet, *Patients' Rights*, available in a range of minority languages, which provides a summary of an individual's rights and responsibilities in the Health Service.

The leaflet *Patients' Rights* is available from local CHCs, or by sending a stamped and addressed envelope to:

Association of Community Health Councils
30 Drayton Park
London N5 1 PB
Tel: 0171 609 8405 Fax: 0171 700 1152

College of Health
St Margaret's House
21 Old Ford Road
London E2 9PL
Tel: 0181 983 1225 Fax: 0181 983 1553
National Waiting List Helpline: 0181 983 1133
(10am to 5pm Monday to Friday)

The College aims to help people prevent ill health and to provide advice on self-care when ill, finding the best treatment and making the best use of the NHS. It produces a number of useful guides.

Genetic Interest Group (GIG)
Farringdon Point
29-35 Farringdon Road
London EC1M 3JB
Tel: 0171 430 0090 Fax: 0171 430 0092

GIG is a source of information and education about genetic disorders. For information about local groups and publications contact the above address.

Pain Relief Foundation
Rice Lane
Liverpool L9 1AE
Tel: 0151 523 1486 Fax: 0151 521 6155

The Foundation has published a substantial body of literature about pain and its treatment, primarily for professionals. In addition they have available a series of eight leaflets on different kinds of chronic pain and a good general guide:

In Pain? A self-help guide for chronic pain sufferers. Price: £8.49 inc p+p.

Visitors are welcome by appointment.

The Patients' Association
8 Guilford Street
London WC1N 1DT
Tel: 0171 242 3460 Fax: 0171 242 3461

An independent charity, which offers advice to individual patients and carers on patients' rights, complaints procedures, and access to health services and appropriate self-help groups.

Complementary and Alternative Medicine

There is no umbrella organisation for complementary and alternative medicine as each therapy has its own regulatory body. Whilst the addresses below will provide some information to point you in the right direction, they cannot provide lists of practitioners.

Council for Complementary Medicine
179 Gloucester Place, London NW1 6DX

Institute for Complementary Medicine
P.O Box 194, London SE16 1QZ

British Holistic Medical Association
Trust House, Royal Shrewsbury Hospital South
Mytton Oak Road
Shrewsbury SY3 8XF

British Complementary Medicine Association
St Charles Hospital
Exmoor Street, London W10 6DZ

ALZHEIMER'S DISEASE

Alzheimer's Disease Society
Gordon House
10 Greencoat Place
London SW1P 1PH
Tel: 0181 306 0606
Fax: 0181 306 0808

ATAXIA

Ataxia
Copse Edge
Thursley
Elstead
Godalming
Surrey GU8 6DJ

ATAXIA TELANGIECTASIA

Ataxia Telangiectasia Society
33 Tuffnells Way
Harpenden
Herts AL5 3HA
Tel: 01582 761437

CEREBRAL PALSY

SCOPE
12 Park Crescent
London W1N 4EQ
Tel: 0171 636 5020
Fax: 0171 436 2601

SOS (Stars Organisation Supporting action for people with Cerebral Palsy)
Wakes Hall
Wakes Colne
Colchester CO6 2DB
Tel: 01787 222044
Fax: 01787 222649

CHARCOT MARIE TOOTH DISEASE

Charcot Marie Tooth International
121 Lavernock Road
Penarth,
South Glamorgan
CF64 3QG
Tel: 01222 709537

DEAFNESS AND HEARING LOSS

Hearing Concern - The British Association of the Hard of Hearing
7-11 Armstrong Road
London W3 7JL
Tel: 0181 743 1110
(voice and text)
Fax: 0181 742 9043

National Deaf Children's Society
15 Dufferin Street
London ECIY 8PD
Tel: 0171 250 0123
(voice and text)
Fax: 0171 251 5020

RNID - The Royal National Institute for Deaf People
19-23 Featherstone St
London ECIY 8SL
Tel: 0171 296 8000
Fax: 0171 296 8199
Textphone:
0171 296 8001

Sense, The National Deafblind and Rubella Association
11/13 Clifton Terrace
London N4 3SR
Tel: 0171 272 7774
Fax: 0171 272 6012
Textphone:
0171 272 9648

DYSPHASIA

Action for Dysphasic Adults (ADA)
Canterbury House
1 Royal Street
London SE1 7LN
Tel. 0171 261 9572

DYSTONIA

The Dystonia Society
Weddel House
13 - 14 West Smithfield
London EC1A 9HY
Tel: 0171 329 0797
Fax: 0171 329 0689

EPILEPSY

British Epilepsy Association
Anstey House
40 Hanover Square
Leeds LS3 1BE
Tel: 0113 243 9393
Fax: 0113 242 8804
Free Helpline:
0800 309 030

Epilepsy Association of Scotland
48 Govan Road
Glasgow G51 1JL
Tel: 0141 427 4911
Fax: 0141 427 7414

The National Society for Epilepsy
Chalfont St Peter
Bucks SL9 0RJ
Tel: 01494 873991
Fax: 01494 871927

FRIEDREICH'S ATAXIA - SEE ATAXIA

GUILLAIN-BARRÉ SYNDROME

Guillain-Barré Syndrome Support Group
Lincolnshire County Council, Council Offices
Eastgate,
Sleaford
Lincoln NG34 7EB
Tel: 01529 304615
Fax: 01529 304615

HUNTINGTON'S DISEASE

Huntington's Disease Association
108 Battersea High Street
London SW11 3HP
Tel: 0171 223 7000
Fax: 0171 223 9489

Scottish Huntington's Association
Thistle House
61 Main Road
Elderslie,
Johnstone
Strathclyde PA5 9BA
Tel: 01505 322 245
Fax: 01505 382 980

INCONTINENCE

The Continence Foundation
2 Doughty Street
London WC1N 2PH
Tel: 0171 404 6875
Fax: 0171 404 6876
Helpline: 0191 213 0050
(Mon to Fri, 9 am - 6pm)

LEARNING DISABILITIES

MENCAP - Royal Society for Mentally Handicapped Children and Adults
Mencap National Centre
123 Golden Lane
London EC1Y 0RT
Tel: 0171 454 0454
Fax: 0171 608 3254

ENABLE
(Scottish Society for the Mentally Handicapped)
6th Floor, 7 Buchanan St
Glasgow GI 3HL
Tel: 0141 226 4541
Fax: 0141 204 4398

People First (London Boroughs)
Instrument House
207/215 Kings Cross Rd
London WC1X 9DB
Tel: 0171 713 6400
Fax: 0171 833 1880

Meningitis

The Meningitis Trust
Fern House
Bath Road
Stroud
Gloucestershire GL5 3TJ
Tel: 01453 751 738
(voice and text)
Fax: 01435 753 588
Helpline (24 hours):
0345 538118

Mental health

MIND (National Association for Mental Health)
Granta House
15/19 Broadway
London E15 4BQ
Tel: 0181 522 2122,
Fax: 0181 522 1725
Information line:
0181 522 1728

National Black Mental Health Association
c/o Rochford Trust
70 Grand Parade
Green Lanes
London N4 1DU
Tel & Fax: 0181 800 2039

Scottish Association for Mental Health
Atlantic House
38 Gardner's Crescent
Edinburgh EH3 8DQ
Tel: 0131 229 9687
or 0131 228 5185
Fax: 0131 229 3558

Motor neurone disease

Motor Neurone Disease Association
PO Box 246
Northampton NN1 2PR
Tel: 01604 250 505
or 01604 22269
Fax: 01604 24726
Helpline: 0345 626 262
(local rates)

Scottish Motor Neurone Disease Association
50 Parnie Street
Glasgow G1 5LS
Tel: 0141 945 1077

Multiple sclerosis

Multiple Sclerosis Society of Great Britain and Northern Ireland
25 Effie Road
London SW6 1EE
Tel: 0171 610 7171
Fax: 0171 736 9861
Helpline: 0171 371 8000

Muscular dystrophy

Muscular Dystrophy Group of Great Britain and Northern Ireland
7/11 Prescott Place
London SW4 6BS
Tel: 0171 720 8055
Fax: 0171 498 0670

Myalgic encephalomyelitis

Action for ME and Chronic Fatigue
PO Box 1302
Wells
Somerset BA5 2WE
Tel: 01749 670 799
Fax: 01749 672 561
Counselling line: 01749 670 402

Myalgic Encephalomyelitis Association
Stanhope House
High Street
Stanford-le-Hope,
Essex, SS17 0HA
Tel: 01375 642 466
Fax: 01375 360 256
Office closed between 12.30 and 1.30pm

Myasthenia gravis

Myasthenia Gravis Association
Keynesa House
77 Nottingham Road
Derby DE1 3QS
Tel: 01332 290219
Fax: 01332 293641

Neurofibromatosis

The Neurofibromatosis Association
Head Office
82 London Road
Kingston-upon-Thames
Surrey BT61 3HP
Tel: 0181 547 1636

Pain

Pain Association Scotland
Cramond House
Kirk Cramond
Cramond Glebe Road
Edinburgh EH4 6NS
Tel: 0131 312 7955

The Pain Relief Foundation
Rice Lane
Liverpool L9 1AE

Pain-Wise UK
33 Kingsdown Park
Takerton
Kent CT5 2DT

Parkinson's disease

Parkinson's Disease Society of the UK
22 Upper Woburn Place
London WC1H 0RA
Tel: 0171 383 3513
Fax: 0171 383 5754

Progressive supranuclear palsy

The Progressive Supranuclear Palsy (PSP Europe) Association
The Old Factory
Wappenham nr Towcester
Northamptonshire
NN12 8SQ
Tel: 01327 860342
Fax: 01327 860242

Rare conditions

Contact a Family
170 Tottenham Court Rd
London W1P 0HA
Tel: 0171 383 3555
Fax: 0171 383 0259

RTMDC (Research Trust for Metabolic Diseases in Children)
Golden Gates Lodge
Weston Road
Crewe,
Cheshire CW2 5XN
Tel: 01270 250 221
Fax: 01270 250 244

Rett syndrome

UK Rett Syndrome Association
29 Carlton Road
London N11 3EX
Tel: 0181 361 5161

Speech impairment

AFASIC (Association For All Speech Impaired Children)
347 Central Markets
Smithfield
London EC1A 9NH
Tel: 0171 236 3632/6487
Fax: 0171 236 8115

Stroke

The Stroke Association
CHSA House
Whitecross Street
London EC1Y 8JJ
Tel: 0171 490 7999
Fax: 0171 490 2686

Tuberous sclerosis

Tuberous Sclerosis Association
Little Barnsley Farm
Catshill,
Bromsgrove
Worcs B61 0NQ
Tel: 01527 871898

Health Publications

The CaF Directory of Specific Conditions and Rare Syndromes in Children with their Family Support Networks, published by Contact a Family (CaF). The CaF Directory provides information on conditions and syndromes that is often difficult to find, even in medical textbooks. The information is very clearly written and includes details of self-help and support groups, regional Genetics Centres, children's hospices and Respite Care Units and other helpful organisations.

Available from:
Contact a Family
16 Strutton Ground
London SW1P 2HP
Tel: 0171 383 3555. Price: £56.00 plus £4.00p+p (subscription for two updates a year £15.00 pa).

The Health Address Book, published by the Patients' Association. Lists over 1000 voluntary organisations, including many self-help groups, concerned with a wide range of disabilities and health problems.

Available from:
The Patients' Association
8 Guilford Street
London WC1N 1DT
Tel: 0171 242 3460 Fax: 0171 242 3461

Community Service Volunteers
237 Pentonville Road
London N1 9NJ
Tel: 0171 278 6601 Fax: 0171 837 9621

The CSV places young people (between 16 and 35) as full-time volunteers in settings throughout the UK to assist people where their help is needed. Many of the placements are in community care settings and each placement will usually last between 4 and 12 months.

CSVs offer a flexible form of help which is responsive to the needs of the people who use it. Many work with individuals on Independent Living Projects, where they can help in various aspects of daily life, including personal care, practical tasks and access to leisure, work and other activities.

People using CSVs provide the volunteer with accommodation, board, travelling expenses and pocket money.

Caring

Association of Crossroads Care Attendant Schemes Ltd
10 Regent Place
Rugby
Warwickshire CV21 2PN
Tel: 01788 573 653 Fax: 01788 565 498

The key objective of this Association is to relieve the stresses experienced by carers and avoid the circumstances which lead to breakdowns and possible admission to hospital or residential care.

The Association promotes the establishment of community-based care attendant schemes.

The schemes are managed by local voluntary committees and staffed by trained co-ordinators and care attendants who work flexibly to provide personal assistance in a way that is homely and complementary to the efforts of other individuals and services involved within the home.

Carers National Association
20/25 Glasshouse Yard
London EC1A 4JS
Tel: 0171 490 8818 Fax: 0171 490 8824
Carers' Line: 0171 490 8898

With a national network of over 100 branches, Carers National Association aims to develop appropriate support for carers, including bringing the needs of carers to the attention of policy makers. It provides information to carers and professionals who work with carers, and aims to encourage carers to recognise their own needs.

All enquirers to the service receive an individual response from an adviser/counsellor.

Carers National Association has produced an excellent series of factsheets and leaflets. Membership costs £3.00 pa, and all members receive a bimonthly newsletter. A publications list is available.

LINGUISTIC SUPPORT

Language Line is a service which offers translation services and telephone conferencing to the health service, police and business users, on the basis of an annual subscription from the organisation using it.

Language Line
18 Victoria Park Square
London E2 9PF
Tel: 0181 983 4042

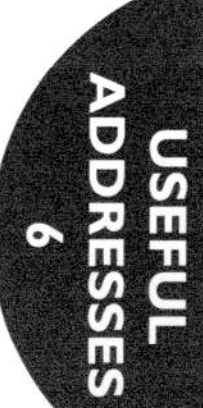

Children and families

Contact a Family
170 Tottenham Court Road
London WI P OHA
Tel: 0171 383 3555 Fax: 0171 383 0269

CaF has a detailed knowledge of both national and local groups acting on behalf of children, publishes relevant information, and has a *Directory of Specific Conditions and Rare Syndromes with their Family Support Networks* (see page 199 for details).

Council for Disabled Children
National Children's Bureau
8 Wakley Street
London ECIV 7QC
Tel: 0171 843 6000

The Council for Disabled Children is devoted to the development of services for disabled children and their families and the exploration of relevant policy issues.

The National Deaf Children's Society
15 Dufferin Street
London ECIY 8PD
Tel: 0171 250 0123 (voice and text)
Fax: 0171 251 5020
Family Freephone (1 am - 5 pm): 0800 252 380

The society provides a range of services including independent and impartial advice and guidance on all aspects of childhood deafness.

Advisory Centre for Education (ACE) Ltd
1B Aberdeen Studios
22-24 Highbury Grove
London N5 2DQ
Tel: 0171 354 8318 Fax: 0171 354 9069
Telephone Advice Line: 0171 354 8321
(2pm to 5pm, Monday to Friday)

ACE aims to assist people to be more involved in education and to make effective choices. It promotes greater consideration of the views of parents and students in educational decisions.

As well as publishing information on issues important to parents, students and teaching professionals, ACE runs a free telephone advice line and produces a number of very useful publications.

Telephone enquiries to the advice line are welcome between 2pm and 5pm Monday to Friday.

Centre for Studies on Inclusive Education
1 Redland Close
Elm Lane, Redland
Bristol BS6 6UE
Tel: 0117 923 8450 Fax: 0117 923 8460

CSIE aims to raise public, professional and political awareness of the issues of integration. It exchanges information relating to integration.

IPSEA Independent Panel for Special Education Advice
22 Warren Hill Road
Woodbridge
Suffolk IP12 4DU
Tel: 01394 382 814 Fax: 01394 380 518

IPSEA offers parents an expert second opinion on the educational needs of their children. (These will generally be children who have been, or are being, assessed under the provisions of the 1993 Education Act).

Expert opinions come from a voluntary panel of qualified professionals, experienced in the field of special education.

The National Association for Special Education Needs (NASEN)
4 - 5 Amber Business Village
Amber Close
Tamworth
Staffordshire B77 4RP
Tel: 01827 311 500 Fax: 01827 313 005

NASEN exists to promote the development of children and young people with special educational needs, wherever they are located, and to support those who work with them. A list of publications and courses produced by NASEN is available from: NASEN Enterprises Ltd., 2 Lichfield Road, Stafford ST17 4JX. Tel: 01785 46872 Fax: 01785 41187.

Network 81
1-7 Woodfield Terrace,
Stansted
Essex CM24 8AJ
Helpline: 01279 647 415
Fax: 01279 816 438

Network 81 co-ordinates a national network of parents of children with special educational needs. Telephone enquiries are welcome between 10 am and 2pm Monday to Friday.

Skill
The National Bureau for Students with Disabilities
336 Brixton Road
London SW9 7AA
Tel: 0171 274 0565 (voice and text)
Fax: 0171 274 7840
Information line: 0171 978 9890 (voice and text)

Skill aims to develop opportunities for people with disabilities and learning difficulties in further, higher and adult education, training and employment throughout the UK. It also has an information service and many publications for students, staff and parents. A network of regional groups throughout the UK is organised as part of the membership scheme.

Telephone enquiries are welcome between 2pm and 4pm Monday to Friday. Visitors are welcome by appointment.

Money

- Local CABs, DIALs and Debt Advice Centres provide advice on benefits, allowances, and financial problems.
- Benefits Agency (an executive agency of the DSS) Benefit Enquiry Lines:
  - ~ for disabled people:
    England, Scotland and Wales: Tel: 0800 882 200
    Northern Ireland: Tel: 0800 220 674
  - ~ for deaf/hearing impaired people.
    Tel: 0800 243 355
  - ~ in languages other than English:
    Urdu:Tel: 0800 289 188
    Chinese:Tel: 0800 252 451
    Punjabi:Tel: 0800 521 360
    Welsh:Tel: 0800 289 011

These lines have been set up to provide information and to assist disabled people to apply for any of the benefits to which they may be entitled. A forms completion service is available on: 0800 441 144.

A translation service is available in over 140 languages.

The Disability Alliance Educational and Research Association
Universal House
88-94 Wentworth Street
London El 7SA
Tel: 0171 247 8776 (voice and text)
Fax: 0171 247 8765

Telephone Benefits Rights Advice Line
Tel: 0171 247 8763 (voice and text)

Publishes a number of helpful guides.

Sex and personal relationships

Relate. Marriage Guidance
Herbert Gray College
Little Church Street
Rugby CV21 3AP
Tel: 01788 573 241 Fax: 01788 535 007

Relate operates in England, Northern Ireland and Wales. Its services are available to those in marriage or other personal relationships. Counselling normally takes place in Relate premises. Some counsellors have specialist knowledge of disability.

Appointments to see a Relate counsellor can be made by telephoning, visiting or writing to the nearest Relate office, details of which can be found under Marriage Guidance or Relate in local telephone directories.

SPOD: Association to Aid the Sexual and Personal Relationships of People with a Disability
286 Camden Road
London N7 OBJ
Tel: 0171 607 8851

SPOD provides information on disability and sexuality, including a range of publications.

Women

Maternity Alliance
45 Beech Street
London EC2P 2LX
Tel: 0171 588 8582 Fax: 0171 588 8584
Textphone: 0171 588 8583

The Alliance works to improve rights and services for mothers, fathers, and babies in the first year of their lives. There is a Disability Working Group, and relevant information is available for disabled people about pregnancy and early parenthood.

Women's Health
52 Featherstone Street
London ECIY 8RT
Tel: 0171 251 6580 Fax: 0171 608 0928

This organisation provides information on a wide range of topics to help women to make informed decisions about their health.

Publication: *Women and Disability* by Susan Lonsdale (Macmillan Press Ltd, 1990). This book draws on interviews with 22 women of different ages, races and socio-economic backgrounds, all of whom have experienced physical or sensory disability which had not arisen out of a natural process of ageing. It looks at the significance of disability for a woman's self-image, and its impact on her sexuality, relationships, marriage and childrearing, and considers how gender-related discrimination can limit independence. Employment policies, the financial consequences of disability, and civil rights are critically examined, and the book concludes positively by examining routes to greater independence and self-determination.

Available from Macmillan Press Ltd., Houndmills, Basingstoke, Hampshire RG21 2XS. Price: £10.99.

AIDS AND EQUIPMENT

In general, local social services departments supply aids, equipment and adaptations to assist a disabled person with daily living. However, these may not be provided free of charge and some local authorities may require the disabled person to be means tested

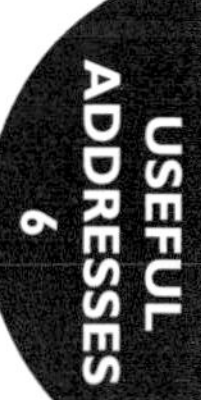

before equipment is supplied. Unfortunately, the level and range of free provision of aids and equipment can vary from one local authority to another.

The National Health Service will provide some aids and items of equipment required for medical care at home. These include back rests, bed cradles, bed pans, commodes, crutches, hoists, mattresses, plastic sheets and walking frames. GPs have a list of items that are available from the local health authority and may also be able to recommend the prescription of items not listed.

Note that section 4 of the Disabled Persons (Services, Consultation and Representation) Act 1986 allows disabled people or carers to ask for an assessment of their needs and that Section 47 of the National Health Service and Community Care Act 1990 requires local authorities, without necessarily being requested to do so, to assess the care needs of people who in its view may require community care services. In assessing the needs of disabled people, the authority must inform them of their rights, and then decide on their need for services. They may, if necessary, liaise with and seek the assistance of relevant health and housing authorities.

Disabled Living Centres There is a network of over 30 Disabled Living Centres in the United Kingdom, providing an equipment exhibition/demonstration and information service to disabled people, carers and professionals concerned with care provision. Most of the centres have a broad range of information covering aspects of daily living.

The centres employ trained staff who offer impartial advice, enabling visitors to make informed decisions about aids, adaptations and services. Training on a wide variety of subjects related to daily living is available to disabled people, carers and professionals.

Disabled Living Centres are located in many towns throughout Britain. To find out the address of your nearest one, you can contact:

The Disabled Living Centres Council
Ist floor, Winchester House
11 Cranmer Road, London SW9 6EJ
Tel: 0171 820 0567 Fax: 0171 735 0278

Communication Aids Centres (CACs) offer assessment, advice and training in the use of communication aids. They are most frequently located in hospitals and the usual way to visit a centre is by referral from a speech and language therapist.

However, this does not prohibit someone contacting their nearest centre directly.

CACs are located in the following towns:

Belfast	Tel: 01232 669 501 Ext. 2917
Birmingham	Tel: 0121 627 8235
Bristol	Tel: 0117 970 1212 Ext. 2151 or 2145
Cardiff	Tel: 01222 566 281 Ext. 3708
Edinburgh EH8	Tel: 0131 667 1438
Edinburgh EH11	Tel: 0131 313 1656
Glasgow	Tel: 0141 649 4545 Ext. 5579/80
Leicester	Tel: 0116 251 6811
Lewes	Tel: 01825 722 112
Lincoln	Tel: 01522 512 512
London WC1	Tel: 0171 837 7618
London W6	Tel: 0181 846 1057/8
London SW3	Tel: 0181 846 6488
London SE7	Tel: 0181 316 7589

Newcastle upon Tyne	Tel: 0191 233 1567
Oldham	Tel: 0161 627 0363
Oxford	Tel: 01865 63508
Sheffield	Tel: 0114 276 6555 Ext. 127
Southampton	Tel: 01703 796 455
Truro	Tel: 01872 74242 Ext. 2470

If you have difficulty in finding a local CAC, contact:
The College of Speech and Language Therapists
7 Bath Place, Rivington Street
London EC2A 3DR
Tel: 0171 613 3855 Fax: 0171 613 3854

Purpose-designed equipment
REMAP GB
Technical Equipment for Disabled People
Hazeldene, Ightham, Sevenoaks
Kent TN15 9AD
Tel: 01732 883 818

Through over 100 local panels, REMAP will make every attempt to solve problems which have not been overcome by standard equipment. Engineers, with the advice of medical and paramedical professionals, will design and make equipment to suit the disabled individual.

REMAP's work is voluntary. The REMAP Yearbook contains information on equipment which has been designed and produced to meet a disabled person's need. The Yearbook also includes the addresses of local panels. It can be obtained from the national organiser at the address above. Price £3.00 inc p+p.

Equipment for short-term loan The Red Cross Medical Loan Service can provide urgently needed equipment such as wheelchairs and commodes on shortterm loan, either for home or holiday use.

Details of the nearest loan service depot can be found in the local telephone directory.

Retail suppliers of aids and equipment Some chemists stock a limited range of aids, and there are a few disability equipment shops in some parts of the country (see your Yellow Pages). The following business offers wider product ranges:

Alfred Bekker
Kellythorpe Industrial Estate
near Driffield
East Yorkshire Y025 9DJ
Tel: 01377 241 700 Fax: 01377 241 767

Alfred Bekker has a shopping centre stocking a very wide range of aids, including wheelchairs, scooters, and equipment for kitchens and bathrooms.

Driving

The Department of Transport (DoT) Mobility Unit offers information and advice on all aspects of transport, both public and private, for people with disability.

Department of Transport Mobility Unit,
Zone 1/11
Greatminster House
76 Marsham Street
London SW1P 4DR
Tel: 0171 271 5257

The DoT also runs a Mobility Advice and Vehicle Information Service (MAVIS) which offers advice, information and assessment facilities for disabled and elderly drivers. They also produce *A Guide to Services in the UK* (new edition, November 1996) which lists all the accredited assessment centres in the UK, and details their facilities.

Department of Transport
Mobility Advice and Information Service
O Wing
Macadam House
Old Wokingham Road
Crowthorne
Berks RG45 6XD
Tel: 01344 661000 Fax: 01344 661066

Disabled people may access assessment centres either directly themselves, or via a health care professional, usually a GP or physiotherapist. The largest centre in the UK is at Banstead in Surrey. This offers assessment facilities for both wheelchairs and driven vehicles.

Banstead Mobility Centre
Damson Way
Orchard Hill
Queen Mary's Avenue
Carshalton
Surrey SM5 4NR
Tel: 0181 770 1151

Vehicles may be leased or hired from Motability, a registered charity which also provides funding, under certain circumstances, for vehicle purchase.

Motability
Goodman House
Station Approach
Harlow
Essex CM20 2ET
Tel: 01279 635 666

There are also various clubs and user groups for disabled drivers throughout the country, with different criteria for eligibility. The largest of these is:

The Disabled Driver's Association
Ashwellthorpe
Norwich NR16 1EX

Local sources of support

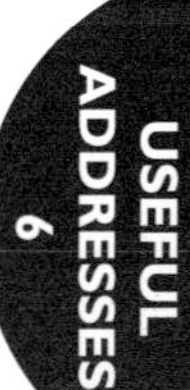

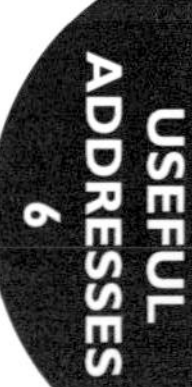
USEFUL ADDRESSES
6

INDEX